CRQs for the Final FRCA

CRQs for the Final FRCA

Caroline Whymark
Consultant in Anaesthesia and Pain Medicine,
University Hospital Crosshouse,
NHS Ayrshire and Arran, UK

Ross Junkin
Consultant in Anaesthesia,
University Hospital Crosshouse,
NHS Ayrshire and Arran, UK

Judith Ramsey
Consultant in Anaesthesia and Intensive Care Medicine,
University Hospital Crosshouse,
NHS Ayrshire and Arran, UK

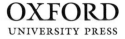

OXFORD
UNIVERSITY PRESS

OXFORD
UNIVERSITY PRESS

Great Clarendon Street, Oxford, OX2 6DP,
United Kingdom

Oxford University Press is a department of the University of Oxford.
It furthers the University's objective of excellence in research, scholarship,
and education by publishing worldwide. Oxford is a registered trade mark of
Oxford University Press in the UK and in certain other countries

© Oxford University Press 2021

First Edition Published in 2021

Impression: 1

Published in the United States of America by Oxford University Press
198 Madison Avenue, New York, NY 10016, United States of America

British Library Cataloguing in Publication Data

Data available

Library of Congress Control Number: 2020951318

ISBN 978-0-19-885030-4

DOI: 10.1093/oso/9780198850304.001.0001

Printed and bound by
CPI Group (UK) Ltd, Croydon, CR0 4YY

Preface

Principles of CRQs in The Final FRCA Exam

This exam preparation book is for the Final Fellowship of the Royal College of Anaesthetists (FRCA) written exam and focuses solely on the Constructed Response Question (CRQ). This exam paper is commonly used to measure knowledge and application-level cognitive skills. CRQs were introduced as a modernization of the Final FRCA written paper in September 2019, replacing 6 of the 12 previous Short Answer Questions (SAQs). By the following year, it replaces these SAQs entirely. The questions will continue to be marked out of 20 and the paper will have a duration of 3 hours (15 minutes per question).

The theory behind this change is to both direct and limit the response of the candidate to answering only the specific question being asked. This promotes a focusing of effort to point-scoring areas of the topic and enhanced time management in this long, arduous paper. In using a more structured question template, the ability of the examiners to deliver a more reliable, reproducible, and valid mark scheme is facilitated. These are features typical of a CRQ:

- Open-ended SAQs with precise answer templates
- Can include 'real world' information (scenarios, cases, investigation results, images)
- Consisting of around 3–6 subsections
- Subsections increasing in complexity and difficulty as the question progresses
- Most commonly used to measure both knowledge and application-level cognitive skills, not simply factual recall

Multiple reasons for candidates failing the Final FRCA have been cited. The 2 main reasons candidates score poorly in this written exam are:

- Failing to answer the specific question asked
- Failing to take heed of the marks' weighting, distributed across the subsections

Additionally, a lack of clinical experience is apparent in some candidates' answers. It is possible that training programme structure may not have allowed a candidate time to complete the relevant training rotations in the subspecialities in which they are examined. The problem of sitting the exam too early is now mitigated by the extended window to achieve the FRCA being pushed back into ST5.

Historically, the SAQs tended to ask a clinical question with multiple aspects of the topic to be addressed for a total of 20 marks. Originally, it was not clear how the marks were allocated throughout the question. Thus candidates could write too much in an area where there were actually few marks, leaving them less time to write an adequate answer in areas worth more marks. Subsequent exam changes led to each SAQ becoming fragmented into 2–4 separate parts, each with the number of marks stated for that specific part. This was to provide a strong hint of how candidates should divide their time more appropriately. However, with unlimited space in answer booklets, candidates continued to make the cardinal error of spending a large volume of time/detail on subsections of good individual knowledge, despite the availability of minimal marks, and to the detriment of answering the whole paper. Better time management would have allowed gaining the easy marks in the remainder of the SAQs where the breadth of knowledge required to pass the FRCA is demonstrated.

The transition from SAQ to CRQ can be thought of as moving further along the continuum, away from the open-ended essay of old, towards an increased structure and mandated response. Gone are the days of the examiner throwing out a net, unsure of what will come back. The enhanced structure brings benefits to both candidate and examiner. A structured exam means a structured mark scheme which is easier to mark. This reduces variation and increases validity with the ultimate goal of ensuring that the good candidates are reliably most likely to pass. The CRQ brings all this together. The question (20 marks) is split into around 3–6 subsections, each showing the number of marks available as before. In addition, there will be a finite space provided to write the answer in. This will guide the candidate in how much they are expected to write. Further, where a list is required, candidates should look for instances of instruction, e.g. 'List the causes of X (4 marks)' may now be 'List 4 causes of X (4 marks)' and 4 lines will actually be provided. This will physically prevent candidates from writing excessively on their favourite or best-known topics.

Finally, the enduring problem of handwriting in exams has been considered. The old adage 'if they can't read it, they can't score it' has been a cause of lost marks to some more than others. Computer-based examining is consistent with the principles of CRQs and appears to be the natural direction of travel for this exam.

Disclaimer

The content of this book is the result of a mixture of compiled clinical experience, author opinion, allied expert opinion, best practice guidance and up-to-date evidence base as practised in the UK per date of publication. The topics considered in the exam questions were intentionally chosen by the authors to reflect a full spectrum of the Final FRCA curriculum. The exam candidate must make a judgement in providing a correct answer. Clearly there will be instances of differing opinion given the often-encountered clinical contention and the authors are fully accepting of this fact. Hence the authors have simply provided a 'proposed answer' given the clinical information described. Answers are accompanied by links to further reading.

The content of this book relates to the Curriculum for a CCT in Anaesthetics 2010 (update v1.8 August 2017) which is examined in the Final FRCA (http://www.rcoa.ac.uk). It does not reflect the views of the RCoA, nor has it been endorsed by it.

The authors and publishers do not accept responsibility or legal liability for any recommendations, errors in the text, or for the misuse or misapplication of material in this work. Medical knowledge and practice is updated continually. This book is designed to provide accurate authoritative information about the subject matter in question. However, readers are advised to check the most current information available and consider this alongside the variations which do occur in local practice throughout the UK. It is the responsibility of the practitioner to take all appropriate safety precautions and clinical liability.

Contents

Abbreviations

ACh	acetylcholine receptor
ACT	acceptance and commitment therapy
AF	atrial fibrillation
AIP	acute intermittent porphyria
APLS	advanced paediatric life support
ARDS	acute respiratory distress syndrome
ASA	American Society of Anesthesiologists
AVF	arteriovenous fistula
BET	bolus/elimination/transfer
BMI	body mass index
CKD	chronic kidney disease
CNS	central nervous system
COPD	chronic obstructive pulmonary disease
CPAP	continuous positive airway pressure
CRPS	complex regional pain syndrome
CRQ	Constructed Response Question
CSHA	Canadian Study of Health and Ageing
CT	computed tomography
CVP	central venous pressure
CXR	Chest X-ray
DIEP	deep inferior epigastric perforator
ED	emergency department
ENT	ears, nose, throat
ET	endotracheal tube
FRC	functional residual capacity
FRCA	Fellowship of the Royal College of Anaesthetists
GBS	Guillain-Barré syndrome
GCS	Glasgow Coma Scale
GFR	glomerular filtration rate
HDU	high dependency unit
IABP	intra-aortic balloon pump
IASP	International Association for Study of Pain
ICU	intensive care unit
IPH	inadvertent perioperative hypothermia
LMA	laryngeal mask airway
LV	left ventricle

MABP	mean arterial blood pressure
MAC	maximum aerobic capacity
MAD	mucosal atomization device
MCH	mean cell haemoglobin
MCV	mean cell volume
MH	malignant hyperthermia
NDMR	non-depolarizing muscle relaxants
OCP	oral contraceptive pill
OME	oral morphine equivalent
ORIF	open reduction and internal fixation
OSA	obstructive sleep apnoea
PCA	patient controlled analgesia
PEEP	positive end-expiratory pressure
POCD	postoperative cognitive dysfunction
RASS	Richmond Agitation-Sedation Scale
RCoA	Royal College of Anaesthetists
RSI	rapid sequence intubation
TAP	transversus abdominus plane
TCI	target-controlled infusion
TIA	transient ischaemic attack
TIVA	total intravenous anaesthesia
TN	trigeminal neuralgia
TSAT	transferrin saturation
VF	ventricular fibrillation
VT	ventricular tachycardia
WFNS	World Federation of Neurosurgeons Scale

Introduction

This book

This book contains 6 practice exam papers, each comprising 12 CRQs. The content is the result of a mixture of compiled clinical experience, author opinion, allied expert opinion, best practice guidance, and up-to-date evidence base as practised in the UK as per date of publication. The topics considered in the exam questions were intentionally chosen to represent the full spectrum of the Final FRCA curriculum. The exam candidate must make a judgement in providing a correct answer. Clearly there will be instances of differing opinion given the often-encountered clinical contention. We, the authors, are fully accepting of this fact hence we have provided a 'suggested answer' given the clinical information described. Most answers contain intentional redundancy, providing some reasonable leeway for the candidate (i.e. there are frequent instances of supernumerary answers provided, more than are required for full marks). Clearly the answers provided are not 'encyclopaedic' in their remit but are weighted towards the more common or clinically relevant in UK medicine. This is both practical and intentional. Answers are accompanied by links to further reading where appropriate.

Final FRCA curriculum—units of training

The Final FRCA exam tests the candidate's knowledge of both the basic and intermediate curricula set out by the Royal College of Anaesthetists, UK. Each written paper will contain 6 CRQs from general duties (which may include a maximum of 1 question from the optional units of training) and 1 CRQ from each of the 6 mandatory units of training. Advanced sciences and professionalism in medicine may be included in any of the questions. The units of training are listed in Table 0.1.

Curriculum changes

At the time of writing the anaesthesia curriculum is undergoing a major rewrite. All postgraduate curricula must meet the standards set out by the General Medical Council (GMC)'s *Excellence by design*. We have anticipated a formalized unit of training in perioperative medicine, preoperative assessment, and prehabilitation and have included questions from these emerging areas. It is hoped the changes to structure of training will also allow more candidates to have gained direct clinical experience of all of the clinical areas in which they are being examined.

Tips

Each question is referenced. Some contain additional tips or pertinent facts not included in the 20 marks available. This means the questions remain a realistic size with an appropriate volume of content and are intended to aid further revision rather than as optional extras to add into the exam answer. Marks should not be awarded for answers not in the mark scheme.

Table 0.1 FRCA units of training

General duties	Mandatory units
1. Airway management 2. Critical incidents 3. Day surgery 4. General, urological, and gynaecological surgery 5. ENT, maxillofacial, and dental surgery 6. Management of respiratory and cardiac arrest 7. Non-theatre 8. Orthopaedic surgery 9. Perioperative medicine 10. Regional anaesthesia 11. Sedation 12. Transfer medicine 13. Trauma and stabilization	1. Anaesthesia for neurosurgery, neuroradiology, and neurocritical care 2. Cardiothoracic anaesthesia and cardiothoracic critical care 3. Intensive care medicine 4. Obstetric anaesthesia 5. Paediatric anaesthesia 6. Pain medicine

Optional units	Advanced sciences
1. Ophthalmic anaesthesia 2. Plastics and burns 3. Vascular surgery anaesthesia	1. Anatomy 2. Applied clinical pharmacology 3. Applied physiology and biochemistry 4. Nutrition 5. Physics and clinical measurement 6. Statistical basis for trial management 7. Professionalism of medical practice

Reproduced with permission from the Royal College of Anaesthetists.

Exam practice

The subject matter will not be unfamiliar to the well-prepared candidate. The critical skills to practice are reading the exact detail of each question, appreciating mark weightings, selecting what to write, and managing time. We suggest the practice questions be attempted under exam conditions with strict time limits in place; 15 minutes per question or 3 hours per 12 question paper and without any significant preconsideration. While we recommend undertaking the questions under exam conditions, some candidates may instead prefer to examine individual curriculum topics to supplement their private study. To facilitate this, our questions are also grouped together by curriculum topic in Appendix 1. Some questions are attributable to multiple units of training.

Role, experience, and affiliation

We are each UK-based NHS Consultant Anaesthetists and Fellows of the Royal College of Anaesthetists (RCoA) with College Tutor experience. We have ongoing commitments to teaching and exam preparation in our region. We have no affiliation with the RCoA's examinations department and have no input into, or knowledge of, their discussions and decisions around any aspect of fellowship exams.

We have peer-reviewed, double-checked, and cross-referenced this manuscript more times than can be counted but inevitably there may be errors. Some of our purported answers may be considered contentious due to differences of opinion or as medicine and clinical practice evolve and change. We are fully accepting of this. Our answers reflect the most recent guidance available at the time of submission of this manuscript. Printed medium becomes quickly outdated in the digital world.

We wish all future candidates well with their preparation and ultimately, success in the Final FRCA exam.

Exam 1 **Questions**

Exam 1 contains 12 selected Constructed Response Questions (CRQs) balanced across the intermediate curriculum, reflecting the Final Fellowship of the Royal College of Anaesthesia (FRCA) exam. We recommend attempting these questions under exam conditions. Please limit/contain your answer to/within the dotted lines given for each question.

Question 1

You are asked to review a 23-year-old primigravida. A lower limb postpartum neurological deficit is suspected. She is 24 hours post-delivery of a 3.9kg baby. She had a forceps delivery in theatre under epidural top-up anaesthesia.

A. List 2 obstetric features which are commonly associated with postpartum neurological deficits (2 marks)

1. ....

2. ....

B. Define the following terms with respect to nerve injury (3 marks)

Nerve injury	Definition
Neuropraxia (1 mark)	
Axonotmesis (1 mark)	
Neurotmesis (1 mark)	

C. Describe the clinical features of the following nerve palsies (12 marks)

Nerve affected	Common mechanism of injury (4 marks)	Sensory and motor deficits (8 marks)
Lateral cutaneous nerve of thigh	1.	1. .... 2. ....
Obturator nerve	1.	1. .... 2. ....
Common peroneal nerve	1.	1. .... 2. ....
Femoral nerve	1.	1. .... 2. ....

D. List the 3 features suggestive of epidural abscess (1 mark)

1. ....

2. ....

3. ....

E. What are the priorities in management of a suspected epidural abscess? (2 marks)

1. ....

2. ....

Total 20 marks

Question 2

A nurse on the intensive care unit (ICU) has asked you to review a 69-year-old man. He is currently intubated as part of the management of an episode of urosepsis. He had been improving over the last 24 hours. However, he has now become restless and agitated. He has no history of alcohol excess but smokes 20 cigarettes a day.

A. Define delirium (1 mark)

....

....

B. Briefly describe 2 different presentations of delirium (2 marks)

1. ....

2. ....

C. List 4 patient risk factors for delirium (4 marks)

1. ....

2. ....

3. ....

4. ....

D. List 2 iatrogenic risk factors for delirium associated with hospital admission (2 marks)

1. ....

2. ....

E. What scoring systems can be used to diagnose delirium in the ICU? (2 marks)

1. ....

2. ....

F. List the 4 components of the CAM-ICU delirium screening tool (4 marks)

1. ....

2. ....

3. ....

4. ....

G. You are investigating and treating the patient's underlying medical problems.

List the non-pharmacological (3 marks) and pharmacological (2 marks) options for treating this patient's delirium.

Non-pharmacological

1. ....

2. ....

3. ....

Pharmacological

1. ....

2. ....

Total 20 marks

Question 3

A 79-year-old man requires transurethral resection of prostate (TURP) for benign prostatic hyperplasia. He has a history of chronic obstructive pulmonary disease (COPD) and angina.

A. What are the advantages of recommending spinal anaesthesia in this case? (3 marks)

1. ....

2. ....

3. ....

B. a) What is the most commonly used irrigation fluid for TURP surgery in the UK? (1 mark)

....

b) Briefly describe 2 properties of this fluid which are not ideal? (2 marks)

1. ....

2. ....

C. List 5 features of an ideal bladder irrigation fluid for use during TURP (5 marks)

1. ....

2. ....

3. ....

4. ....

5. ....

D. The patient becomes unwell during surgery. You suspect TURP syndrome

What features of established TURP syndrome may be apparent? (4 marks)

CNS (2 marks)	1. ....
	2. ....
CVS (2 marks)	1. ....
	2. ....

E. You check the patient's urea and electrolytes. What is the most likely biochemical abnormality? (1 mark)

....

F. Describe 4 measures which are in place to reduce the incidence of TURP syndrome in theatre (4 marks)

1. ....

2. ....

3. ....

4. ....

Total 20 marks

Question 4

A 75-year-old man with type 2 diabetes presents to day surgery for elective inguinal hernia repair. He takes metformin and gliclazide daily, and Lantus 80u at night. He also takes enalapril for hypertension and has a glyceryl trinitrate (GTN) spray that he uses a few times per week.

A. List the general criteria that a patient must meet to have surgery as a day case (3 marks)

1. ....

2. ....

3. ....

B. List the criteria specific to this patient that must be met for day case surgery (3 marks)

1. ....

2. ....

3. ....

C. Give 3 surgical considerations for the operation to be done as day case surgery (3 marks)

1. ....

2. ....

3. ....

D. His HbA1c was last checked 2 weeks earlier and was 75mmol/L (9%)

a) What does this value represent at a cellular level? (1 mark)

b) What does this process represent at a clinical level? (1 mark)

c) How long does it take to see any change in HbA1c? Why is this? (1 mark)

E. Should his surgery proceed? State why (2 marks)

Please answer Yes or No next and give one reason to support your answer.

F. List 2 pros and 2 cons of a spinal anaesthetic for this type of patient? (2 marks)

Pros

1.

2.

Cons

1.

2.

G. How would you manage his diabetes in the preoperative period? Give specific advice regarding medication (4 marks)

1. ....

2. ....

3. ....

4. ....

Total 20 marks

Question 5

A 37-year-old female presents to the emergency department with sudden onset of headache. Computed tomography (CT) head indicates subarachnoid haemorrhage (SAH). You are asked to review the patient and on examination find their eyes closed, moaning and groaning, and withdrawing from pain. There is no obvious motor deficit. Pupils are equal and reactive.

A. What is the patient's Glasgow Coma Scale (GCS) (1 mark), and the SAH grade according to the World Federation of Neurosurgeons Scale (WFNS)? (1 mark)

....

....

B. List 5 indications for tracheal intubation following acute SAH (5 marks)

1. ....

2. ....

3. ....

4. ....

5. ....

C. The patient is transferred to a neurosurgical unit. A subsequent CT angiogram reveals a wide-necked aneurysm in the Circle of Willis. Name the arteries in the Circle of Willis figure here (5 marks)

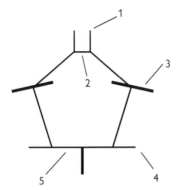

1. ....

2. ....

3. ....

4. ....

5. ....

D. The patient has a craniotomy for clipping of aneurysm and recovers well; 4 days later she develops a new hemiparesis. What is the definition of a delayed neurological deficit (DND)? (1 mark)

....

....

E. List 4 complications which may contribute to DND? (4 marks)

1. ....

2. ....

3. ....

4. ....

F. In the neurosurgical ICU, the patient's mean arterial blood pressure is 82mmHg and intracranial pressure is 12mmHg. Calculate the cerebral perfusion pressure (1 mark)

G. What therapies are available to improve cerebral blood flow due to vasospasm following SAH? (2 marks)

Total 20 marks

Question 6

You are allocated to deliver anaesthesia for electroconvulsive therapy (ECT). The list is located in the psychiatry unit.

A. What is the definition of remote site anaesthesia? (2 marks)

B. Briefly describe 3 main goals of anaesthetic technique specific to ECT? (3 marks)

1.

2.

3.

C. Describe the cardiovascular response to ECT? (5 marks)

1. ....

2. ....

3. ....

4. ....

5. ....

D. How can seizure activity be altered by anaesthetic technique? (4 marks)

1. ....

2. ....

3. ....

4. ....

E. Describe the role of muscle relaxation during ECT? Include an example (2 marks).

1. ....

2. ....

F. A 73-year-old woman is pre-assessed for consideration of possible ECT. Her medical history is severe depression. Her current drug history includes phenelzine. What class of drug is phenelzine? (2 marks)

1. ....

2. ....

G. Describe the clinical significance of phenelzine to anaesthesia (2 marks)

....

....

....

....

Total 20 marks

Question 7

A 76-year-old lady presents to the preoperative assessment clinic prior to a right total hip replacement. The nursing staff are concerned regarding her frailty.

A. What are the 2 main models to describe frailty? (2 marks)

1. ....

2. ....

B. What are the risk factors for frailty? (9 marks)

1. ....

2. ....

3. ....

4. ....

5. ....

6. ....

7. ....

8. ....

9. ....

C. Give an example of a tool that can be used to assess frailty? (1 mark)

....

....

D. What is prehabilitation? (2 marks)

....

....

....

E. What are the 4 main components of the multimodal approach to prehabilitation? (4 marks)

1. ....

2. ....

3. ....

4. ....

F. What are the potential outcome benefits of prehabilitation? (2 marks)

1. ....

2. ....

Total 20 marks

Question 8

A 64-year-old man has refractory left ventricular failure following a myocardial infarction. The next step in his management is to insert an intra-aortic balloon pump (IABP).

A. Describe the principles of using an IABP (4 marks)

....

....

....

....

B. Complete the table that follows, listing the haemodynamic effects of an IABP on the aorta, heart, and coronary blood flow (6 marks)

	Haemodynamic effects
Aorta (2 marks)	1. .... 2. ....
Heart (3 marks)	1. .... 2. .... 3. ....
Coronary artery blood flow (1 mark)	1. ....

C. List 4 contraindications to IABP insertion (4 marks)

1. ....

2. ....

3. ....

4. ....

D. List 6 early complications of IABP insertion (6 marks)

1. ....

2. ....

3. ....

4. ....

5. ....

6. ....

Total 20 marks

Question 9

A 26-year-old lady breaks her ankle dancing in a nightclub. She has open reduction and internal fixation of fibula the following day which proceeds uneventfully.

At review 16 weeks later, she reports persisting severe pain in the ankle. The orthopaedic surgeon queries complex regional pain syndrome (CRPS) and refers her to the pain clinic.

A. What is the definition of CRPS? (3 marks)

....

....

....

....

B. List the signs and symptoms associated with CRPS (4 marks)

	Signs/ Symptoms
Sensory (1 mark)	
Motor (1 mark)	
Sudomotor (1 mark)	
Vasomotor (1 mark)	

C. What are the criteria required for diagnosis of CRPS? (5 marks)

1. ....

2. ....

3. ....

4. ....

5. ....

D. Briefly describe 4 principles of management of CRPS (8 marks)

1. ....

....

2. ....

....

3 ....

....

4. ....

....

Total 20 marks

Question 10

A 2-month-old baby is listed for pyloromyotomy. He was born at term gestation by spontaneous vaginal delivery. He has no other significant medical history.

A. List 4 common clinical features of paediatric pyloric stenosis (4 marks)

1. ....

2. ....

3. ....

4. ....

B. State the classic electrolyte imbalance (1 mark) and briefly describe its pathophysiology (2 marks)

....

....

....

....

C. What are the priorities for preoperative optimization? (3 marks)

1. ....

2. ....

3. ....

D. List 5 important anatomical features in the airway of a child of this age (5 marks)

1. ....

2. ....

3. ....

4. ....

5. ....

E. Briefly describe the steps required to induce anaesthesia in this patient in the anaesthetic room? (4 marks)

1. ....

2. ....

3. ....

4. ....

F. What postoperative monitoring is required? (1 mark)

....

Total 20 marks

Question 11

A 74-year-old female patient requires open reduction and internal fixation (ORIF) for fractured shaft of humerus. She takes morphine for arthritis and you decide to perform a brachial plexus block.

A. She is concerned about having a needle near her neck. Give 4 general principles required for consent to be informed (4 marks)

1. ....

2. ....

3. ....

4. ....

B. What is the best approach to the brachial plexus for arm surgery such as this? Give a reason for your answer (3 marks)

....

....

....

C. List 4 precautions you would take to ensure safe and accurate placement of the block before beginning the procedure (4 marks)

1. ....

2. ....

3. ....

4. ....

D. What are the advantages of ultrasound-guided blocks compared to the traditional nerve stimulator approach? (5 marks)

1. ....

2. ....

3. ....

4. ....

5. ....

E. On the diagram to follow, please label the following (3 marks)

   a) inferior trunk
   b) median nerve
   c) medial cord

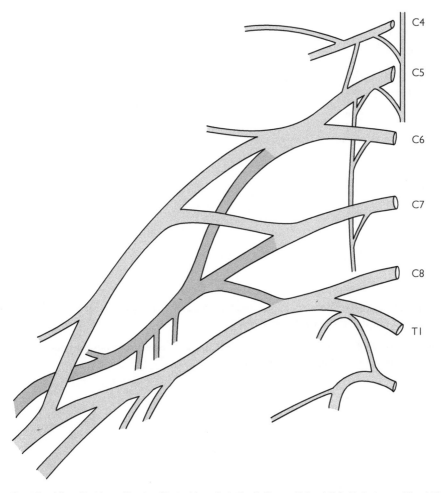

C4

C5

C6

C7

C8

T1

F. Which nerve is most commonly damaged in the perioperative period? (1 mark)

....

Total 20 marks

Question 12

A 32-year-old woman requires temporomandibular joint (TMJ) arthrocentesis under general anaesthesia. She has no other significant medical history.

A. What are the symptoms of TMJ dysfunction? (4 marks)

1. ....

2. ....

3. ....

4. ....

B. On preoperative assessment the patient has mouth opening measured at 2cm. You plan a fibreoptic intubation (FOI) via the nasal route.

What factors would influence whether the nasal FOI was undertaken with the patient awake or under general anaesthesia? (6 marks)

	Factors
Awake FOI (3 marks)	1. .... 2. .... 3. ....
Asleep FOI (3 marks)	1. .... 2. .... 3. ....

C. Describe what premedication may be considered to improve the subsequent intubating conditions, include examples (3 marks)

1. ....

2. ....

3. ....

D. You induce general anaesthesia and the patient's mouth opening does not improve following muscle paralysis. Describe a detailed stepwise technique of asleep FOI via the nasal route (7 marks)

1. ....

2. ....

3. ....

4. ....

5. ....

6. ....

7. ....

Total 20 marks

Exam 1 **Answers**

Many of the following questions contain more answers than there are marks allocated. This redundancy is intentional and is to ensure that a spread of possible answers by the candidate are recognized. 1 mark is awarded per correct point up to the maximum specified in each subsection.

Question 1

You are asked to review a 23-year-old primigravida. A lower limb postpartum neurological deficit is suspected. She is 24 hours post-delivery of a 3.9kg baby. She had a forceps delivery in theatre under epidural top-up anaesthesia.

A. List 2 obstetric features which are commonly associated with postpartum neurological deficits
   (2 marks)

   1. Primigravida
   2. Prolonged second stage
   3. Assisted delivery including forceps and caesarean
   4. Foetal macrosomia   (2)

   Note: Do not accept anaesthesia-related features (e.g. regional anaesthesia) as the question asks for obstetrics. Also, anaesthesia-related nerve injuries are less common.

B. Define the following terms with respect to nerve injury (3 marks)

Nerve injury	Definition
Neuropraxia (1 mark)	Temporary and physiological interruption of conduction without loss of axonal continuity
Axonotmesis (1 mark)	Loss of the relative continuity of the axon and its covering of myelin, but preservation of the connective tissue framework of the nerve
Neurotmesis (1 mark)	Total severance or disruption of the entire nerve fibre with no distal nerve conduction

(3)

C. Describe the clinical features of the following nerve palsies (12 marks)

Nerve affected	Common mechanism of injury (4 marks)	Sensory and motor deficits (8 marks)
Lateral cutaneous nerve of thigh	1. Compression with thigh flexion as it passes under the inguinal ligament, worsened by the pregnant abdomen	1. Sensory—anterolateral thigh 2. Motor—nil
Obturator nerve	2. Compression by the foetal head during descent or during forceps delivery	3. Sensory—inner thigh 4. Motor—weakness of hip adduction (crossing legs)
Common peroneal nerve	3. Compression at neck of fibula such as by stirrups in lithotomy position	5. Sensory—lateral lower leg and dorsum of foot 6. Motor—foot drop
Femoral nerve	4. Compression against inguinal canal during forceps or caesarean	7. Sensory—anterior thigh, absent knee jerk 8. Motor—weakness of knee extension/difficulty climbing stairs

(12)

D. List the 3 features suggestive of an epidural abscess (1 mark)

1. Pain—back pain or radicular pain
2. Sepsis—raised inflammatory markers, constitutional upset
3. Neurology—lower limb weakness and/or urinary/anal dysfunction

Note: All 3 required for 1 mark (1)

E. What are the priorities in management of a suspected epidural abscess? (2 marks)

1. Expedite urgent MRI lumbar spine
2. Discuss with neurosurgical registrar
3. Discuss with senior anaesthetist (2)

Total marks 20

Further reading

H Boyce, F Plaat; Post-natal neurological problems, *Continuing Education in Anaesthesia Critical Care & Pain*, Volume 13, Issue 2, 1 April 2013, Pages 63–66.

Question 2

A nurse on the ICU has asked you to review a 69-year-old man. He is currently intubated as part of the management of an episode of urosepsis. He had been improving over the last 24 hours however he has now become restless and agitated. He has no history of alcohol excess but smokes 20 cigarettes a day.

A. **Define delirium** (1 mark)

An acute disturbance in cognitive function OR a disturbance in consciousness and cognition that develops over a short period of time   (1)

B. **Briefly describe 2 different presentations of delirium** (2 marks)

1. Hyperactive—agitation, aggression, hallucinations, and restlessness
2. Hypoactive—inattention, decreased awareness of surroundings, motor retardation, apathy, can appear sedated
3. Or can be fluctuating between the 2   (2)

C. **List 4 patient risk factors for delirium** (4 marks)

1. Increasing age
2. Pre-existing cognitive impairment/dementia
3. Visual/hearing impairment
4. Alcohol abuse
5. Hypertension
6. Depression
7. Smoking   (4)

D. **List 2 iatrogenic risk factors for delirium associated with hospital admission** (2 marks)

1. Medications, e.g. benzodiazepines, anticholinergics
2. Sleep disturbance
3. Immobilization
4. Unfamiliar circumstances; moving wards, change of staff in shift patterns   (2)

E. **What scoring systems can be used to diagnose delirium in the ICU?** (2 marks)

1. CAM-ICU (confusion assessment method for the ICU) assessment of delirium symptoms
2. ICDSC—Intensive Care Delirium Screening Checklist—which combines assessment of sedation and delirium to give a score
3. An agitation/sedation scoring system such as RASS (Richmond Agitation-Sedation Scale) or Riker Sedation-Agitation Scale.   (2)

F. List the 4 components of the CAM-ICU delirium screening tool (4 marks)

1. Acute onset of mental status changes or a fluctuating course, AND
2. Inattention, AND
3. Disorganized thinking, OR
4. Altered level of consciousness = DELIRIUM   (4)

Data from Ely EW, Margolin R, et. al. Evaluation of delirium in critically ill patients: validation of the Confusion Assessment Method for the Intensive Care Unit (CAM-ICU). *Crit Care Med.* 2001 Jul;29(7):1370–9.

G. You are investigating and treating the patient's underlying medical problems. List the non-pharmacological (3 marks) and pharmacological (2 marks) options for treating this patient's delirium

Non-pharmacological

1. Sleep/wake correction—re-establish diurnal pattern
2. Sedation holds/breaks
3. Orientation
4. Use of hearing/visual aids
5. Physiotherapy and mobilization   (3)

Pharmacological

1. Haloperidol is the first line drug treatment
2. Antipsychotic such as olanzapine
3. Nicotine patch as heavy smoker   (2)

Note: No marks given for benzodiazepines. These should generally be avoided for delirium except in acute alcohol withdrawal.

Total 20 marks

Further reading

J King, A Gratrix; Delirium in intensive care, *Continuing Education in Anaesthesia Critical Care & Pain*, Volume 9, Issue 5, 1 October 2009, Pages 144–147.

Question 3

A 79-year-old man requires TURP for benign prostatic hyperplasia. He has a history of COPD and angina.

A. What are the advantages of recommending spinal anaesthesia in this case? (3 marks)

1. May be preferable for patients with significant respiratory disease
2. Good postoperative analgesia
3. Reduced stress response to surgery
4. Allows monitoring of conscious level and early detection of TURP syndrome
5. Reduced blood loss   (3)

B. a) What is the most commonly used irrigation fluid for TURP surgery in the UK? (1 mark)

    1. Glycine 1.5%   (1)

  b) Briefly describe 2 properties of this fluid which are not ideal? (2 marks)

    1. Hypotonic (220mosmol/kg) with respect to plasma (280–300mosmol/kg)

    2. Metabolically active as a neurotransmitter—can precipitate direct CNS toxicity and generates ammonia as a metabolite   (2)

C. List 5 features of an ideal bladder irrigation fluid for use during TURP (5 marks)

    1. Transparent for good visibility

    2. Electrically non-conductive

    3. Isotonic

    4. Non-toxic/inert

    5. Non-haemolytic when absorbed

    6. Sterile

    7. Long shelf life

    8. Inexpensive   (5)

D. The patient becomes unwell during surgery. You suspect TURP syndrome. What features of established TURP syndrome may be apparent? (4 marks)

CNS (2 marks)	1. Headache 2. Altered conscious level (including coma) 3. Seizures 4. Visual disturbance
CVS (2 marks)	1. Pulmonary oedema/cardiac failure/fluid overload 2. Myocardial ischaemia

                                                      (4)

E. You check the patient's urea and electrolytes. What is the most likely biochemical abnormality? (1 mark)

Hyponatraemia   (1)

Note: caused by rapid absorption of a large volume of hypotonic irrigation fluid.

F. Describe 4 measures which are in place to reduce the incidence of TURP syndrome in theatre (4 marks)

    1. Height of irrigation fluid above the patient should be kept to a minimum (usually 60–70cm)

    2. Avoiding prolonged surgery (>1h)

    3. Avoiding bladder perforation—allows a large volume of fluid into the peritoneal cavity where it is absorbed

4. Surgical technique—laser prostatectomy and vaporization techniques generally cause less bleeding and less absorption of fluid into open veins

5. Avoiding low venous pressure in the patient (4)

Total 20 marks

Further reading

AM O'Donnell, ITH Foo; Anaesthesia for transurethral resection of the prostate, *Continuing Education in Anaesthesia Critical Care & Pain*, Volume 9, Issue 3, 2009, Pages 92–96.

Question 4

A 75-year-old man with type 2 diabetes presents to day surgery for elective inguinal hernia repair. He takes metformin and gliclazide daily, and Lantus 80u at night. He also takes enalapril for hypertension and a GTN spray that he uses a few times per week.

A. **List the general criteria that a patient must meet to have surgery as a day case** (3 marks)

1. Informed consent to go home the same day
2. Understanding of post-op instructions
3. Responsible adult at home with the patient for 24 hours
4. Access to telephone and transport
5. Lives less than 30 minutes' drive from hospital (3)

B. **List the criteria specific to this patient that must be met for day case surgery** (3 marks)

1. No recent hypoglycaemic attacks
2. Patient and caregiver can monitor blood glucose, interpret, and act upon result
3. HbA1c <9% (75mmol/L)
4. No recent change in angina nature or frequency
5. No recent changes to hypertensive medication

Note: no marks for criteria repeated in both question parts A and B. (3)

Note: neither age nor body mass index (BMI) are specific contraindications to day surgery

C. **Give 3 surgical considerations for operation to be done as day case surgery** (3 marks)

1. Procedure lasts less than 1 hour
2. Simple uncomplicated hernia (no re-do, bowel resection)
3. Minimally invasive technique to be used
4. Ideally placed first on the morning list (3)

D. **His HbA1c was last checked 2 weeks before and was 75mmol/L (9%)**

a) **What does this value represent at a cellular level?** (1 mark)

The HbA1c test measures the proportion of haemoglobin glycosylation in the blood (chemically bonded with glucose) (1)

b) What does this process represent at a clinical level? (1 mark)

It means that blood glucose control has been suboptimal over the preceding 3 months (1)

c) How long does it take to see any change in HbA1c? Why is this? (1 mark)

3 months. This is because glycosylation is an irreversible process. 120 days is the lifespan of erythrocytes (1)

E. Should his surgery proceed? State why (2 marks)

Please answer Yes or No next and give one reason to support your answer.

Answer NO: AAGBI guidelines state to postpone if HbA1c >69mmol/mol (8.5%)

Answer YES: Need to wait 3 months for red cell turnover to see any improvement (2)

F. List 2 pros and 2 cons of a spinal anaesthetic for this type of patient? (2 marks)

Pros

1. Reduced nausea or vomiting
2. Earlier resumption of oral intake including medication
3. Reduced risk of confusion/delirium
4. Facilitates monitoring of cerebration and blood glucose/early alert of hypos

Cons

1. Need a high block to cover peritoneum
2. May worsen cardiac instability or ischaemia
3. May be difficult to site/may not work/inadequate anaesthesia
4. May persist for longer than required prolonging stay

Note: 2 reasons in each category for both marks (2)

G. How would you manage his diabetes in the preoperative period? (4 marks)

Give specific advice regarding medication.

1. Take metformin as usual
2. Do not take gliclazide on day of surgery
3. Take a reduced dose of Lantus night before surgery
4. Allow clear glucose solution to be taken orally if impending hypoglycaemia
5. Monitor blood sugar (4)

Total 20 marks

Further reading

Association of Anaesthetists of Great Britain and Ireland; Peri-operative management of the surgical patient with diabetes 2015, *Anaesthesia*, Volume 70, 2015, Pages 1427–144.

J Canet, J Raeder, LS Rasmussen, et al.; Cognitive dysfunction after minor surgery in the elderly, *Acta Anaesthesiologica Scandinavica*, Volume 47, 2003, Pages 1204–1210.

R Verma, R Alladi, I Jackson, et al.; Day case and short stay surgery: 2, *Anaesthesia*, Volume 66, 2011, Pages 417–434.

Question 5

A 37-year-old female presents to the emergency department with sudden onset of headache. CT head indicates SAH. You are asked to review the patient and on examination find their eyes closed, moaning and groaning, and withdrawing from pain. There is no obvious motor deficit. Pupils are equal and reactive.

A. What is the patient's GCS (1 mark), and the SAH grade according to the WFNS? (1 mark)

1. GCS is 7–E1 (eyes closed), V2 (incomprehensible sounds), and M4 (withdrawing from pain)
2. The WFNS is grade 4 with or without motor deficit   (2)

B. List 5 indications for tracheal intubation following acute SAH? (5 marks)

1. Unconsciousness (GCS <8)
2. Reduction in GCS of ≥2 points
3. For optimization of oxygenation pO_2 >13kPa
4. For optimization of CO_2 4.0–4.5kPa
5. Controlling seizures
6. Protection of the airway in the absence of laryngeal reflexes
7. Transfer to a neurosurgical centre   (5)

C. The patient is transferred to a neurosurgical unit. A subsequent CT angiogram reveals a wide-necked aneurysm in the Circle of Willis. Name the arteries in the Circle of Willis figure that follows (5 marks)

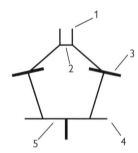

1. Anterior cerebral artery
2. Anterior communicating artery
3. Internal carotid artery
4. Posterior cerebral artery
5. Posterior communicating artery   (5)

D. The patient has a craniotomy for clipping of aneurysm and recovers well, but 4 days later she develops a new hemiparesis. What is the definition of a delayed DND? (1 mark)

DND is any clinically detectable neurological deterioration after initial stabilization, with the exception of re-bleeding. (1)

E. List 4 complications which may contribute to DND? (4 marks)

1. Vasospasm
2. Hydrocephalus
3. Seizures
4. Sepsis/fever
5. Electrolyte abnormality (4)

F. In the neurosurgical ICU, the patient's mean arterial blood pressure is 82mmHg and intracranial pressure is 12mmHg. Calculate the cerebral perfusion pressure? (1 mark)

1. MABP—ICP = CPP
   82–12 = 70mmHg (1)

G. What therapies are available to improve cerebral blood flow due to vasospasm following SAH? (2 marks)

1. Triple H therapy: hypertension, hypervolaemia, haemodilution
2. Calcium channel blockers, e.g. nimodipine
3. Balloon angioplasty/intra-arterial vasodilator, e.g. papaverine (2)

Total 20 marks

Further reading

A Luoma, U Reddy; Acute management of aneurysmal subarachnoid haemorrhage, *Continuing Education in Anaesthesia Critical Care & Pain*, Volume 13, Issue 2, 2013, Pages 52–58.

Question 6

You are allocated to deliver anaesthesia for ECT. The list is located in the psychiatry unit.

A. What is the definition of remote site anaesthesia? (2 marks)

1. The Royal College of Anaesthetists (RCoA) defines a remote site as any location in which an anaesthetist is required to provide general/regional anaesthesia or sedation away from the main theatre suite and/or anaesthetic department
2. It cannot be guaranteed that the help of another anaesthetist will be immediately available
3. This may be either within or away from the base hospital (2)

B. **Briefly describe 3 main goals of anaesthetic technique specific to ECT?** (3 marks)

1. Rapid onset/offset of consciousness with rapid recovery
2. Effective attenuation of the hyperdynamic response to the electrical stimulus
3. Muscle relaxation to prevent injury for the duration of electrical stimulus and subsequent seizure
4. Minimal suppression of seizure activity by the anaesthetic technique (3)

C. **Describe the cardiovascular response to ECT?** (5 marks)

1. Generalized activation of the autonomic nervous system
2. An initial parasympathetic discharge lasting 10–15s. This can result in bradycardia, hypotension, or even asystole
3. A more prominent sympathetic response follows
4. Cardiac arrhythmias occasionally occur during the sympathetic response
5. Systolic arterial pressure may increase by 30–40% and heart rate may increase by 20% or more, generally peaking at 3–5 min
6. Myocardial oxygen consumption increases potentially precipitating ischaemia
7. Systolic and diastolic function can remain decreased up to 6 h after ECT (5)

D. **How can seizure activity be altered by anaesthetic technique?** (4 marks)

1. Intentional hyperventilation to induce hypocapnia may lower seizure threshold and lengthen seizure duration
2. Choice of induction agent—recognition of spectrum of anticonvulsant properties
3. Titration of induction agent dose—modification of dose is informed by the seizure quality during previous ECT treatments
4. Avoidance of premedication
5. Co-administration of other dose-sparing IV induction drugs, e.g. opioids (4)

E. **Describe the role of muscle relaxation during ECT? Include an example** (2 marks)

1. Succinylcholine (0.5mg/kg) is most commonly used
2. Neuromuscular blocking agents reduce muscular convulsions and decrease the risk of serious injury (during unmodified fits, there is a risk of fractures and dislocations but these are now rare)
3. Dental damage and oral cavity lacerations are also described (insert bite protection) (2)

F. **A 73-year-old woman is pre-assessed for consideration of possible ECT. Her medical history is severe depression. Her current drug history includes phenelzine. What class of drug is phenelzine?** (2 marks)

1. Monoamine oxidase inhibitor
2. Non-selective, irreversible (2)

G. Describe the clinical significance of phenelzine to anaesthesia (2 marks)

1. Administration of indirectly acting sympathomimetic agents such as ephedrine or metaraminol should be avoided as these may precipitate a severe hypertensive reaction

2. The next best choice to treat a drop in blood pressure is phenylephrine which is direct acting. Adrenaline and noradrenaline would be safe to use, however due to their potency would not be considered a first line choice (2)

Notes: In general, a cautious approach would be to discontinue monoamine oxidase inhibitors (MAOIs) before ECT if the medication has not been helpful. Risk benefit balance should be discussed with the psychiatry team on an individual case by case basis.

Total 20 marks

Further reading

Z Ding, P White; Anesthesia for electroconvulsive therapy 2002, *Anesthesia & Analgesia*, Volume 94, Issue 5, 2002, Pages 1351–1364.

M Nevin, L Brennan; Anaesthetic services in remote sites, *Royal College of Anaesthetists*, 2014 https://www.rcoa.ac.uk/ document-store/anaesthetic-services-remotesites

V Uppal, J Dourish, A Macfarlane; Anaesthesia for electroconvulsive therapy, *Continuing Education in Anaesthesia Critical Care & Pain*, Volume 10, Issue 6, 2010, Pages 192–196.

Question 7

A 76-year-old lady presents to the preoperative assessment clinic prior to a right total hip replacement. The nursing staff are concerned regarding her frailty.

A. What are the 2 main models to describe frailty? (2 marks)

1. The frailty phenotype
2. The frailty index (2)

B. What are the risk factors for frailty? (9 marks)

1. Advancing age
2. Comorbidities such as cardiovascular disease
3. Diabetes mellitus
4. Stroke/cerebrovascular disease
5. Cancer
6. Arthritis
7. COPD
8. Anaemia
9. Female sex
10. Lower socioeconomic class
11. Depression
12. Disability, or difficulty with activities of daily living (9)

C. Give an example of a tool that can be used to assess frailty? (1 mark)

No standardized method available but examples include:

1. Edmonton Frail Scale
2. Canadian Study of Health and Ageing (CSHA) frailty index   (1)

D. What is prehabilitation? (2 marks)

Prehabilitation is the process of enhancing an individual's functional capacity (1 mark) to enable him/her to withstand a forthcoming stressor, e.g. major surgery (1 mark)   (2)

E. What are the 4 main components of the multimodal approach to prehabilitation? (4 marks)

1. Medical optimization
2. Physical exercise
3. Nutritional support
4. Psychological support   (4)

F. What are the potential outcome benefits of prehabilitation? (2 marks)

1. Reduced length of stay
2. Less postoperative pain
3. Fewer postoperative complications   (2)

Total 20 marks

Further reading

Frailty Path https://www.frailtypath.co.uk
R Griffiths, M Mehta; Frailty and anaesthesia: what we need to know, *Continuing Education in Anaesthesia Critical Care & Pain*, Volume 14, Issue 6, December 2014, Pages 273–277.

Question 8

A 64-year-old man has refractory left ventricular failure following a myocardial infarction. The next step in his management is to insert an IABP.

A. Describe the principles of using an IABP (4 marks)

1. The balloon sits in the descending aorta
2. It works using counterpulsation
3. Counterpulsation is a term that describes balloon inflation in diastole and deflation in early systole
4. It is synchronized with the electrocardiogram (ECG) or systemic arterial pressure waveform   (4)

B. Complete the table that follows, listing the haemodynamic effects of an IABP on the aorta, heart, and coronary blood flow (6 marks)

Aorta (2 marks)	1. Decreased systolic pressure 2. Increased diastolic pressure
Heart (3 marks)	1. Decreased afterload 2. Decreased preload 3. Increased cardiac output
Coronary blood flow (1 mark)	1. Increased coronary blood flow/perfusion

(6)

C. List 4 contraindications to IABP insertion (4 marks)

1. Aortic regurgitation
2. Aortic dissection
3. Chronic end-stage heart disease with no anticipation of recovery
4. Aortic stents
5. Uncontrolled sepsis
6. Abdominal aortic aneurysm
7. Tachyarrhythmias
8. Severe peripheral vascular disease
9. Major arterial reconstruction surgery

(4)

D. List 6 early complications of IABP insertion (6 marks)

1. De-synchronization with cardiac cycle increasing the work of the heart
2. Limb ischaemia
3. Thromboembolism
4. Compartment syndrome
5. Aortic dissection
6. Local vascular injury
7. Balloon rupture/gas embolus
8. Thrombocytopenia/haemolysis
9. Malpositioning causing cerebral or renal compromise
10. Cardiac tamponade

(6)

Note: No marks given for infection as this is a later complication

Total 20 marks

Further reading

M Krishna, K Zacharowski; Principles of intra-aortic balloon pump counterpulsation, *Continuing Education in Anaesthesia Critical Care & Pain*, Volume 9, Issue 1, February 2009, Pages 24–28.

Question 9

A 26-year-old lady breaks her ankle dancing in a nightclub. She has ORIF of fibula the following day, which proceeds uneventfully.

At review 16 weeks later, she reports persisting severe pain in the ankle. The orthopaedic surgeon queries CRPS and refers her to the pain clinic.

A. **What is the definition of CRPS?** (3 marks)

1. Severe continuous pain in an extremity
2. Accompanied by sensory, vasomotor, sudomotor, motor/trophic changes
3. Pain is restricted to a region, not anatomical or dermatomal
4. Pain is disproportionate to the inciting event (3)

B. **List the signs and symptoms associated with CRPS** (4 marks)

	Signs and symptoms
Sensory (1 mark)	Hyperaesthesia, dysaesthesia, allodynia
Motor (1 mark)	Muscle wasting, weakness, reduced range of movement, tremor
Sudomotor (1 mark)	Oedema or asymmetry in sweat pattern
Vasomotor (1 mark)	Asymmetry of temperature or colour

Note: 1 mark available per box, no marks for duplication of any signs or symptoms. (4)

C. **What are the criteria required for diagnosis of CRPS?** (5 marks)

1. Budapest criteria accepted and validated
2. Patient must have continuing pain disproportionate to inciting event
3. Other possible diagnoses excluded
4. One symptom in each of 3 of the 4 categories
5. One sign in 2 or more categories *at the time of examination* (5)

D. **Briefly describe 4 principles of management of CRPS?** (8 marks—2 marks for each statement)

1. Early referral to a multidisciplinary team to access a range of therapies
2. Patient education: classes and written/web based materials
3. Pain physiotherapy: graded exercise, mirror therapy, desensitization
4. Pharmacological intervention: class of drug appropriate to assumed type or phase of CRPS, e.g. inflammatory/vasomotor or early/late
5. Psychological intervention: for distress and impact of pain. Acceptance and commitment therapy (ACT)

6. Spinal cord stimulation: realistic option for lower limb CRPS only (8)

Note: Treatment with bisphosphonate infusion (e.g. pamidronate) is an option in the early phase of the syndrome.

Total 20 marks

Further reading

KD Bharwani, M Dirckx, FJPM Huygen; Complex regional pain syndrome: diagnosis and treatment, *BJA Education*, Volume 17, Issue 8, August 2017, Pages 262–268.

P Ganty, R Chawla; Complex regional pain syndrome: recent updates, *Continuing Education in Anaesthesia Critical Care & Pain*, Volume 14, Issue 2, April 2014, Pages 79–84.

RN Harden, S Bruehl, RS Perez, et al.; Validation of proposed diagnostic criteria (the 'Budapest Criteria') for complex regional *pain* syndrome, *Pain*, Volume 150, 2010, Pages 268–274.

Question 10

A 2-month-old baby is listed for pyloromyotomy. He was born at term gestation by spontaneous vaginal delivery. He has no other significant medical history.

A. **List 4 common clinical features of paediatric pyloric stenosis?** (4 marks)

1. Increased incidence in male versus female
2. Usually presents in the 2–3rd month of life
3. Projectile vomiting of non-bilious stomach contents
4. Weight loss/failure to thrive
5. Dehydration
6. Palpable 'olive' on abdominal examination (4)

B. **State the classic electrolyte imbalance** (1 mark) **and briefly describe its pathophysiology?** (2 marks)

1. Hypokalaemic, hypochloraemic metabolic alkalosis (1)

Pathophysiology: any 2 of the following:

1. Due to loss of gastric secretions which are high in hydrogen and chloride
2. Dehydration causes aldosterone secretion with resultant sodium and water retention. Aldosterone influences the Na/K exchange increasing potassium lost in the urine and worsening hypokalaemia
3. Alkaline urine is due to bicarbonate excretion (early)
4. Paradoxical acidic urine (late) as plasma volume maintenance becomes the priority and the kidneys instead excrete hydrogen ions in exchange for sodium and water (2)

C. **What are the priorities for preoperative optimization?** (3 marks)

1. Nil by mouth
2. Accurate assessment of degree or percentage dehydration
3. IV fluid and electrolyte replacement
4. Aim for resolution of alkalosis and restore electrolytes to normal range before theatre
5. Senior help available   (3)

Note: pyloric stenosis is a medical emergency, not a surgical emergency, and the patient should be resuscitated before going to theatre.

D. **List 5 important anatomical features in the airway of a child of this age** (5 marks)

1. Large head/prominent occiput
2. Large tongue
3. High anterior larynx, situated at C3–C4 level
4. Epiglottis is long, stiff, and u-shaped
5. Preferential nasal breather
6. Larynx is funnel-shaped/conical
7. The airway is at its narrowest point at the level of the cricoid   (5)

E. **Briefly describe the steps required to induce anaesthesia in this patient in the anaesthetic room?** (4 marks)

1. Requires pre-induction nasogastric (NG) or orogastric tube if not already *in situ* to empty stomach contents
2. Rotate the infant from supine, aspirating in each position (e.g. to left lateral, to prone, to right lateral). Also consider bedside stomach ultrasound for gastric contents
3. IV cannula *in situ*
4. Gas (sevoflurane) or intravenous (propofol 3mg/kg or ketamine 2mg/kg) induction
5. Gentle bag mask ventilation after induction of anaesthesia
6. Muscle relaxation for laryngoscopy reduces the likelihood of regurgitation when instrumenting the airway
7. Intubate with appropriately sized microcuff endotracheal tube (e.g. size 3.0 mm internal diameter)   (4)

F. **What postoperative monitoring is required?** (1 mark)

Continuous saturation monitoring and apnoea monitor for at least 12 hours   (1)

Total 20 marks

Further reading

L Adewale; Anatomy and assessment of the pediatric airway, *Pediatric Anesthesia*, Volume 19 (Suppl.1), 2009, Pages 1–8.

R Craig, A Deeley; Anaesthesia for pyloromyotomy, *BJA Education*, Volume 18, Issue 6, 2018, Pages 173–177.

Question 11

A 74-year-old female patient requires ORIF for fractured shaft of humerus. She takes morphine for arthritis and you decide to perform a brachial plexus block.

A. She is concerned about having a needle near her neck. Give 4 general principles required for consent to be informed (4 marks)

1. Discuss procedure and common side effects
2. Discuss reasonable alternatives including no block
3. Discuss risks in terms the patient can understand
4. Discuss rare but serious risks plus those the patient may consider important (material risks) (4)

B. What is the best approach to the brachial plexus for arm surgery such as this? Give a reason for your answer (3 marks)

1. Supraclavicular approach
2. Most likely block to achieve coverage of the whole operative field
3. Areas of potentially poor block are at the extremes of the plexus and easily accessed for augmentation whereas the humerus is supplied from middle nerve roots (3)

C. List 4 precautions you would take to ensure safe and accurate placement of the block before beginning the procedure (4 marks)

1. Check consent
2. Check correct side for procedure
3. Position the patient with attention to anatomical landmarks
4. Ensure ultrasound available/checked/set up ready to use
5. Avoid sedation
6. STOP before you block (4)

D. What are the advantages of ultrasound-guided blocks compared to the traditional nerve stimulator approach? (5 marks)

1. Direct visualization of nerves, blood vessels, and needle
2. Accuracy of needle placement
3. Rapid block onset
4. Reduced dose of local anaesthetic required
5. Reduced procedural pain
6. Fewer complications
7. Visualization of local anaesthetic spread
8. Avoids stimulation of painful fracture site (5)

E. On the diagram that follows, please label (3 marks)

    a) inferior trunk

    b) median nerve

    c) medial cord

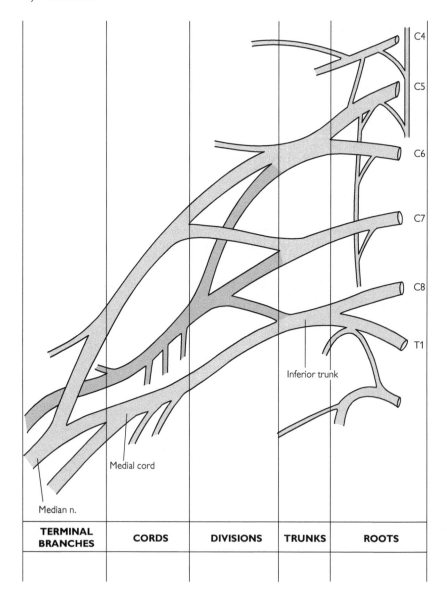

TERMINAL BRANCHES	CORDS	DIVISIONS	TRUNKS	ROOTS

Reproduced from *Principles and Practice of Regional Anaesthesia* (4 ed.), Graeme McLeod, Colin McCartney, and Tony Wildsmith, Figure 17.1. Copyright Oxford University Press, 2012. Reproduced with permission of the Licensor through PLSclear.

(3)

F. Which nerve is most commonly damaged in the perioperative period? (1 mark)

1. Ulnar nerve due to pressure from positioning and immobility.   (1)

Total 20 marks

Further reading

P Kumar, BC Raju, DM Coventry; Ultrasound-guided brachial plexus blocks, *Continuing Education in Anaesthesia Critical Care & Pain*, Volume 14, Issue 4, August 2014, Pages 185–191.

Question 12

A 32-year-old woman requires TMJ arthrocentesis under general anaesthesia. She has no other significant medical history.

A. What are the symptoms of TMJ dysfunction? (4 marks)

1. Pain in one or both TMJs
2. Difficulty chewing/eating
3. Clicking/locking
4. Poor mouth opening
5. Headaches/facial pain   (4)

B. On preoperative assessment the patient has a mouth opening measured at 2cm. You plan a FOI via the nasal route.

What factors would influence whether the nasal FOI was undertaken with the patient awake or under general anaesthesia? (6 marks)

	Factors
Awake FOI (3 marks)	1. Raised BMI 2. Predicted difficulty with mask ventilation 3. Obstructive sleep apnoea 4. Other coexisting airway abnormalities
Asleep FOI (3 marks)	1. Poor patient compliance, uncooperative 2. Fasted 3. No significant reflux 4. Ability to successfully insert oropharyngeal airway is predicted

No marks for repeating opposites.   (6)

C. Describe what premedication may be considered to improve the subsequent intubating conditions, include examples (3 marks)

1. Antisialogogues, e.g. glycopyrrolate 4mcg/kg IM, 1 hour preoperatively to dry secretions

2. Topical vasoconstrictor to nose, e.g. 0.5ml co-phenylcaine spray via mucosal atomization device (MAD) to each nostril or xylometazoline hydrochloride spray (e.g. Otrivine®) to improve nasal passage opening and reduce its vascularity

3. Nebulized epinephrine to improve nasal passage opening and reduce its vascularity

4. Antacid to reduce risk of regurgitation, e.g. H_2 antagonist, proton pump inhibitor   (3)

D. You induce general anaesthesia and the patient's mouth opening does not improve following muscle paralysis. Describe a detailed stepwise technique of asleep FOI via the nasal route (7 marks)

1. Ensure ability to hand ventilate the patient to maintain oxygenation/anaesthesia
2. Operator, patient, and screen are aligned for optimal comfort and scope handling
3. Scope is preloaded with the endotracheal tube, e.g. size 6.0mm internal diameter reinforced or nasal preformed
4. Keep the scope straight
5. Navigate the nose—look through both nostrils with the scope and choose the larger orifice
6. Ensure the scope is smoothly manoeuvred to hover above mucosal surfaces
7. Jaw thrust from an assistant to improve the space at base of tongue
8. Locate epiglottis/place glottis in the centre of the screen
9. Pass the scope into the trachea, keeping it above the carina and railroad the endotracheal tube
10. (Anticlockwise) gentle rotating action of endotracheal tube through the cords
11. Confirm intubation by visualization of the tracheal rings/carina via the endotracheal tube
12. Confirmation by capnography

Any mention of these points within the answer are scored to a maximum of 7.   (7)

Total 20 marks

Further reading

G Aiello, I Metcalf; Anaesthetic implications of temporomandibular joint disease, *Canadian Journal of Anesthesia*, Volume 39, Issue 6, 1992, Pages 610–616.

MD Martin, KJ Wilson, BK Ross, K Souter; Intubation risk factors for temporomandibular joint/facial pain, *Anesthesia Progress*, Volume 54, Issue 3, Fall 2007, Pages 109–114.

Exam 2   **Questions**

Exam 2 contains 12 selected Constructed Response Questions (CRQs) balanced across the intermediate curriculum, reflecting the Final Fellowship of the Royal College of Anaesthesia (FRCA) exam. We recommend attempting these questions under exam conditions. Please limit/contain your answer to/within the dotted lines given for each question.

Question 1

A 23-year-old man is admitted to a surgical high dependency unit (HDU). He has a history of Crohn's disease. He presents with gastrointestinal obstruction. His drug history is regular sulphasalazine and a recent course of prednisolone 40mg daily. He weighs 50kg. He is to have 24 hours of conservative management prior to laparotomy. You attend the ward to assess him preoperatively.

A. Briefly outline how you will assess his fluid balance (4 marks)

1. ....

2. ....

3. ....

4. ....

B. What factors may contribute to this patient's fluid deficit? (4 marks)

1. ....

2. ....

3. ....

4. ....

C. You determine he needs fluid prior to theatre due to his recent losses.

List the 4 categories of fluid replacement to be considered (2 marks)

1. ....

2. ....

3. ....

4. ....

D. What are the guiding principles of fluids required for resuscitation and maintenance? (4 marks)

1. ....

....

....

2. ....

....

....

E. Calculate the volume of maintenance fluid this patient needs in 24 hours (1 mark)

....

F. Prescribe maintenance fluid for him for the first 24 hours (1 mark)

....

....

G. Define the anion gap (2 marks)

....

....

....

H. How may infusing 0.9% saline affect the anion gap? (1 mark)

....

....

....

I. How may infusing Hartmann's solution affect the anion gap? (1 mark)

....

....

....

Total 20 marks

Question 2

You are called to the emergency department for a stand-by call for a collapsed 13-month-old child.

A. Complete this table, including detail specific to this patient, to show how you would prepare for their arrival using the advanced paediatric life support (APLS) guideline WETFLAG (7 marks)

W (1 mark)	
E (1 mark)	
T (1 mark)	
F (1 mark)	
L (1 mark)	
A (1 mark)	
G (1 mark)	

B. What other preparations would you make? (5 marks)

....

....

....

....

....

....

....

C. Fill in the following table with normal ranges for a 1–2-year-old child (3 marks)

Heart rate (1 mark)	
Systolic blood pressure (1 mark)	
Respiratory rate (1 mark)	

D. Define the term neonate (1 mark)

....

....

E. What are the 4 commonest causes of neonatal collapse? (4 marks)

1. ....

2. ....

3. ....

4. ....

Total 20 marks

Question 3

A. Define pain (2 marks)

....

....

B. Complete the table showing the pathophysiology of nociceptive versus neuropathic pain
   (1 mark for each correct answer to a maximum of 6 marks)

	Nociceptive	Neuropathic
Origin		
Triggered by		
Indicative of		
Duration		

C. Give 4 different questionnaires that can be used to assess chronic pain (4 marks)

1. ....

2. ....

3. ....

4. ....

D. Give 4 methods of assessing acute pain (4 marks)

1. ....

2. ....

3. ....

4. ....

E. Give 4 problems with these assessment tools? (4 marks)

1. ....

2. ....

3. ....

4. ....

Total 20 marks

Question 4

A 21-year-old man is listed for dental extractions (UR8, LR8, UL8, LL8) as a day case. His only medical history is von Willebrand's disease (vWD) type 1, associated with easy bruising.

A. Define vWD? (2 marks)

....

....

B. What is the specific role of von Willebrand's Factor? (1 mark)

....

C. Indicate the likely findings on blood testing. In the boxes, enter raised [↑], decreased [↓], or normal [↔] for each parameter (1 mark awarded for each correct pair of answers to a maximum of 3 marks)

	Platelet count	Bleeding time	APTT	PT	Fibrinogen	Factor VIII level
Von Willebrand's disease						

D. The patient attends the preoperative assessment clinic. What logistics, investigations, and specific therapies should be considered prior to presenting for surgery?

Logistics (2 marks)	1. ....
	2. ....
Investigations (2 marks)	1. ....
	2. ....
Specific Therapies (2 marks)	1. ....
	2. ....

E. The patient presents on the day of surgery. Describe the advantages and disadvantages of endotracheal intubation via the nasal route in this patient (3 marks)

	Advantage (1 mark)	**Disadvantages** (2 marks)
Nasal intubation	1.	1. ....
		2. ....

F. How can intra- and postoperative bleeding be minimized during this case? (5 marks)

1. ....

2. ....

3. ....

4. ....

5. ....

Total 20 marks

Question 5

A. What factors must you take into account for consent to be considered 'informed'? (5 marks)

1. ....

2. ....

3. ....

4. ....

5. ....

B. Name 2 acts of parliament which legislate for capacity to consent in the UK (2 marks)

1. ....

2. ....

C. What change to the consent process evolved from the Montgomery versus Lanarkshire Health Board judgement handed down March 2015? (3 marks)

....

....

....

D. What difficulties are there in explaining risks to a patient? (4 marks)

....

....

....

....

E. What is a Caldicott Guardian? (2 marks)

....

....

F. What are the 4 principles of ethical decision-making that must be considered in clinical practice? (4 marks)

1. ....

....

2. ....

....

3. ....

....

4. ....

....

Total 20 marks

Question 6

A 73-year-old man presents with a gangrenous left foot and requires an urgent below-knee amputation. He is known to have peripheral vascular disease, previous CVA, COPD, and stable angina. His current medication includes clopidogrel, ramipril, simvastatin, isosorbide mononitrate. He also takes zomorph 30mg b.d. with sevredol 5mg for breakthrough pain and regular paracetamol for ischaemic limb pain.

A. List 3 risk factors for the development of phantom limb pain postoperatively (3 marks)

1. ....

2. ....

3. ....

B. Outline your management of this patient to treat acute pain and attenuate the likelihood of developing chronic pain following amputation using the subheadings to follow

Preoperative (3 marks)

1. ....

2. ....

3. ....

Intraoperative (3 marks)

1. ....

2. ....

3. ....

Postoperative (5 marks)

1. ....

2. ....

3. ....

4. ....

5. ....

C. Outline the correct process during 'Stop Before You Block' (2 marks)

1. ....

2. ....

D. Give the 2 main branches of the sciatic nerve. Describe the motor response elicited by stimulation of each nerve (4 marks)

Nerve (2 marks)	**Motor response** (2 marks)

Total 20 marks

Question 7

A 68-year-old man is known to have aortic stenosis.

A. List 3 cardinal symptoms of worsening aortic stenosis? (3 marks)

1. ....

2. ....

3. ....

B. What are the 3 most common causes of aortic stenosis? (3 marks)

1. ....

2. ....

3. ....

C. Describe the pathophysiology of worsening aortic stenosis (3 marks)

1. ....

2. ....

3. ....

D. He attends preoperative assessment during workup for consideration of a valve intervention. What are the expected abnormal findings in aortic stenosis? (4 marks)

Clinical examination signs (2 marks)	1. ....
	2. ....
ECG findings (1 mark)	1. ....
CXR findings (1 mark)	1. ....

E. An updated echocardiogram is requested as part of the preoperative assessment. Describe 3 specific measurements on echocardiography indicating severe aortic stenosis? (3 marks)

1. ....

2. ....

3. ....

F. List 3 potential valve interventions for severe symptomatic aortic stenosis? (1 mark)

1. ....

2. ....

3. ....

G. You plan to anaesthetise the patient for valve intervention. What are the cardiovascular goals specific to aortic stenosis for this patient? (3 marks)

1. ....

2. ....

3. ....

Total 20 marks

Question 8

A 59-year-old man is scheduled for an elective lumbar discectomy. At the preassessment clinic the nurse is concerned he may have obstructive sleep apnoea (OSA)

A. Complete the STOP-BANG scoring tool for OSA (8 marks)

S (1 mark)	
T (1 mark)	
O (1 mark)	
P (1 mark)	

B (1 mark)	
A (1 mark)	
N (1 mark)	
G (1 mark)	

B. What are the endocrine (3 marks) and cardiovascular (3 marks) consequences of OSA?

Endocrine (3 marks)

1. ....

2. ....

3. ....

Cardiovascular (3 marks)

1. ....

2. ....

3. ....

C. This patient is investigated and diagnosed with OSA. You intend to use high-flow nasal oxygen therapy for preoxygenation and postoperatively. What are the specifics of high-flow nasal oxygen therapy which confer physiological advantage? (6 marks)

1. ....

2. ....

3. ....

4. ....

5. ....

6. ....

Total 20 marks

Question 9

A 90-year-old woman with a fractured neck of femur is scheduled for operative fixation with a dynamic hip screw. She weighs 45kg. She has atrial fibrillation (AF) and takes digoxin 125µg, warfarin 5mg, and furosemide 20mg daily. Her blood pressure is 150/90mmHg and heart rate is 80 beats per minute.

A. Define frailty syndrome (1 mark)

....

....

....

B. From the information in the question, what underlying comorbidities may have caused her fall? Complete the table with at least one cause in each category (5 marks—1 per column)

CVS	CNS	Metabolic	Global changes with age	Infection

C. Complete the table to show the advantages of general versus advantages of regional anaesthesia in this patient? (6 marks)

	Advantages
General anaesthesia (3 marks)	1. .... 2. .... 3. ....
Regional anaesthesia (3 marks)	1. .... 2. .... 3. ....

D. How would you manage her anticoagulation perioperatively? (3 marks)

E. What formal scoring systems could you use to estimate her risk of morbidity and mortality? (1 mark)

F. List 4 of the variables which increase the risk of mortality at 30 days in the frail population (4 marks)

1.

2.

3.

4.

Total 20 marks

Question 10

In the preassessment clinic, a 62-year-old patient requires hysterectomy for endometrial cancer. She has hypertension, depression, back pain, and fibromyalgia. Her body mass index (BMI) is 45.

She takes lisinopril, sertraline, co-codamol (30/500) 8 tablets per day, oxycodone 40mg b.d., and shortec 10mg for breakthrough pain, which she usually requires twice per day. The gynaecologists do not wish to postpone her operation.

A. Describe the main perioperative pain management issue in this patient (1 mark)

B. How much oral morphine equivalent (OME) does she take in 24 hours? (2 marks)

....

....

C. What specific measures would you take to reduce the impact this has perioperatively?
(4 marks)

1. ....

2. ....

3. ....

4. ....

D. Outline your plan for perioperative analgesia (6 marks)

....

....

....

....

....

....

....

....

....

E. You are called to review her in recovery as she reports severe pain. She is using a standard
patient controlled analgesia (PCA) regime of 1mg morphine bolus with a 5-minute lockout.
Give 2 ways you can increase the efficacy of this PCA? (2 marks)

1. ....

2. ....

F. What other analgesics might you consider at this stage? (1 mark)

....

G. What are your instructions on discharge from recovery? (2 marks)

....

....

H. What other classes of drugs might you prescribe for the postoperative period? (2 marks)

....

....

Total 20 marks

Question 11

You have been called to the emergency department to review a 24-year-old man with a significant traumatic brain injury, following an assault. He has no other injuries.

A. What would be the indications to intubate and ventilate this patient? (8 marks)

1. ....

2. ....

3. ....

4. ....

5. ....

6. ....

7. ....

8. ....

B. You intubate and ventilate the patient successfully with cervical spine stabilization and prepare for transfer. Outline your management to prevent secondary brain injury (6 marks)

1. ....

2. ....

3. ....

4. ....

5. ....

6. ....

7. ....

8. ....

C. What are the 2 recommended values to target to prevent secondary brain injury? (2 marks)

Intracranial pressure (1 mark)	
Cerebral perfusion pressure (1 mark)	

D. The patient is transferred safely to the tertiary neurosurgical centre where they find his intracranial pressure is raised, despite your management.

What further options are there to reduce intracranial pressure? (4 marks)

....

....

....

....

Total 20 marks

Question 12

You are asked to see a 24-year-old woman on the postnatal ward who is 36 hours following a spontaneous vaginal delivery. She had an epidural in labour. She is now complaining of severe headache. You suspect a postdural puncture headache (PDPH).

A. List 6 other possible causes of a headache in this patient (6 marks)

1. ....

2. ....

3. ....

4. ....

5. ....

6. ....

B. Describe the pathophysiology of headache in PDPH (3 marks)

....

....

....

....

....

C. List 5 classical symptoms of PDPH (5 marks)

1. ....

2. ....

3. ....

4. ....

5. ....

D. The patient is also complaining of double vision. Describe a likely cause and specific findings on neurological examination (2 marks)

....

....

....

E. List 3 options for management of postdural puncture headache symptoms (3 marks)

1. ....

2. ....

3. ....

F. What factor has the most impact in reducing the incidence of PDPH associated with lumbar epidural? (1 mark)

....

Total 20 marks

Exam 2 **Answers**

Many of the following questions contain more answers than there are marks allocated. This redundancy is intentional and is to ensure that a spread of possible answers by the candidate are recognized. 1 mark is awarded per correct point up to the maximum specified in each subsection.

Question 1

A 23-year-old man is admitted to surgical HDU. He has a history of Crohn's disease. He presents with gastrointestinal obstruction. His drug history is regular sulphasalazine and a recent course of prednisolone 40mg daily. He weighs 50kg. He is to have 24 hours of conservative management prior to laparotomy. You attend the ward to assess him preoperatively.

A. Briefly outline how you will assess his fluid balance (4 marks)

1. History: how long unwell for, recent intake, vomiting, diarrhoea, thirst?
2. Examination: tongue/mucous membranes, skin turgor, CRT, RR, cold peripheries
3. Observations: fluid chart in/out including urine volumes and measured gastrointestinal (GI) losses, HR, BP
4. Investigations: U + E, FBC, protein, and albumin.

Note: Need at least 2 per category for 1 mark   (4)

B. What factors may contribute to this patient's fluid deficit? (4 marks)

1. GI losses/no oral intake
2. Redistribution losses from extracellular fluid (ECF) to interstitial fluid and bowel lumen
3. Pyrexia increasing evaporative losses
4. Some drug therapy increases fluid losses
5. Inadequate volume fluid prescribed; no account taken of maintenance fluids or preadmission deficits
6. Fluids not administered (lack of patent IV access, delay in prescribing, or between bags)   (4)

C. You determine he needs fluid prior to theatre due to his recent losses. List the 4 categories of fluid replacement to be considered (2 marks)

1. Resuscitation
2. Redistribution
3. Replacement and reassessment
4. Routine (maintenance fluids)   (2)

D. **What are the guiding principles of fluids required for resuscitation and maintenance?** (4 marks)

    1. Resuscitation: replacing extracellular fluid so use crystalloid with composition closest to ECF and that will remain in ECF for as long as possible before redistribution.

    Blood as packed red cells may also be required.
No role for colloids/ starches (increased risk of renal failure and increased mortality).
Suggest Hartmann's solution. (2)

    2. Maintenance: replacing total body water and electrolytes throughout the intracellular, extracellular, and interstitial fluid compartments.

    A balanced crystalloid solution is recommended which will not cause hyper or hyponatraemia.
Sodium and potassium both required at a minimum 1mmol/kg/24 hours maintenance.
Suggest 0.18% saline/4% glucose + 20mmol of potassium per 500ml bag. (2)

E. **Calculate the volume of maintenance fluid this patient needs in 24 hours?** (1 mark)

    50kg. Aim 20–30ml/kg = 1,000–1500ml (1)

F. **Prescribe maintenance fluid for him for the first 24 hours** (1 mark)

    0.18% saline/4% glucose + 20 mmol KCl 500ml bag, 8 hourly for 24hours (1)

G. **Define the anion gap** (2 marks)

    1. The anion gap is the difference between the primary measured cations sodium and potassium, and the primary measured anions chloride and bicarbonate, in serum.

    2. $(Na^+ + K^+) — (Cl^- + HCO_3)$ = anion gap in serum (2)

H. **How may infusing 0.9% saline affect the anion gap?** (1 mark)

    Higher anion gap: a metabolic acidosis can occur causing an increase of unmeasured anions (ketones, lactate, hydrogen) which require buffering by bicarbonate. Reduction in bicarbonate causes an increase in chloride hence hyperchloraemic metabolic acidosis. This can be caused by excess fluid replacement with NaCl (or diarrhoea). (1)

I. **How may infusing Hartmann's solution affect the anion gap?** (1 mark)

    Lower anion gap: Too much Hartmann's solution causes a hypochloraemic metabolic alkalosis due to metabolism of lactate to bicarbonate and compensatory reduction in chloride (as can vomiting with loss of H^+). Albumin concentration is important as if low, there is a compensatory increase in chloride and bicarbonate which reduces the gap. (1)

Total 20 marks

Further reading

NICE Guideline CG174; Intravenous fluid therapy in adults in hospital (and algorithm), updated May 2017
https://www.nice.org.uk/guidance/cg174

A Perner et al.; Hydroxyethyl starch versus Ringers acetate in sepsis, *New England Journal of Medicine*, Volume 367, 2012, Pages 124–134.

H Wesley, MD Self; Balanced crystalloids versus saline in non-critically ill adults, *New England Journal of Medicine*, Volume 378, 2018, Pages 819–828.

Note: Many will find the anion gap questions difficult. In total it is worth 4 marks, therefore do not dwell upon it. The question overall can be passed without these marks.

Question 2

You are called to the emergency department for a stand-by call for a collapsed 13-month-old child.

A. Complete this table, including detail specific to this patient, to show how you would prepare for their arrival using the APLS guideline WETFLAG (7 marks)

W (1 mark)	Weight (Age + 4) × 2 = 10kg (1)
E (1 mark)	Energy for defibrillation 4J/kg = 40J (1)
T (1 mark)	endotracheal tube (ET) (Age/4) + 4 = diameter Age/2 + 12 = length at lips for oral tube Age/2 +15 = length for nasal tube (Any 1 of these 3 for a mark)
F (1 mark)	Fluid –20ml/kg crystalloid bolus (for shock other than trauma or DKA) (1)
L (1 mark)	Lorazepam 0.1ml/kg (1)
A (1 mark)	Adrenaline 0.1ml/kg 1:10,000 (1)
G (1 mark)	Glucose 5ml/kg dextrose 10% (1)

Reproduced with permission from Samuels M. and Wieteska S., *Advanced Paediatric Life Support: A Practical Approach to Emergencies*, 6th Edition, Copyright Advanced Life Support Group and Wiley 2016.

(7)

B. What other preparations would you make? (5 marks)

1. Contact relevant personnel, e.g. paediatric resuscitation team (paediatric consultant/ registrar, anaesthetic consultant, senior emergency department (ED) staff)

Airway and breathing:

2. Bag valve mask with appropriate mask sizes

3. Adjuncts: range of oro/nasopharyngeal airways, LMAs
4. Oxygen source, oxygen box and masks, appropriate oxygen saturation probe
5. Availability of a paediatric ventilator

Circulation:
6. IV/IO access available, BM sticks, blood bottles, and blood culture bottles

Disability and exposure:
7. Prepare drugs—usually intensive care network proforma can be used which has all rapid sequence intubation (RSI) and emergency drug doses for preparation
8. Portable ECHO/ultrasound if available
9. Warming equipment prepared and ready

(5)

C. **Fill in the following table with normal ranges for a 1–2-year-old child** (3 marks)

Heart rate (1 mark)	100–150bpm
Systolic blood pressure (1 mark)	85–95mmHg
Respiratory rate (1 mark)	20–35 breaths/min

(3)

D. **Define the term neonate** (1 mark)

A neonate is a newborn child less than 28 days of age, or of less than 44 weeks postconceptual age

(1)

E. **What are the 4 commonest causes of neonatal collapse?** (4 marks)

1. Infection/sepsis
2. Congenital heart disease
3. Inborn errors of metabolism
4. Non-accidental injury

(4)

Total 20 marks

Further reading

APLS guidelines https://www.resus.org.uk/library/2015-resuscitation-guidelines/paediatric-advanced-life-support

S Playfor; Management of the critically ill child with sepsis, *Continuing Education in Anaesthesia Critical Care & Pain*, Volume 4, Issue 1, 1 February 2004, Pages 12–15.

Question 3

A. **Define pain** (2 marks)

'Pain is an unpleasant sensory and emotional experience associated with actual or potential tissue damage or described in terms of such damage'. (2)

Note: This is the International Association for Study of Pain (IASP) definition of pain. 'What the patient says it is' is a *description* not a definition.

B. **Complete the table showing the pathophysiology of nociceptive versus neuropathic pain** (1 mark for each correct answer to a maximum of 6 marks)

	Nociceptive	**Neuropathic**
Origin	Tissue nociceptors, normal activation	Tissue nociceptors; abnormal activation
Triggered by	Noxious stimuli	Any stimulus; can be spontaneous also
Indicative of	Tissue damage	Nerve dysfunction
Duration	Usually acute (<3months)	Chronic (>3months)

(6)

C. **Give 4 different questionnaires that can be used to assess chronic pain** (4 marks)

All must be multidimensional questionnaires.

1. Brief Pain Inventory
2. McGill Pain Questionnaire
3. LANSS Leeds Assessment Neuropathic symptoms and signs
4. HADS Hospital Anxiety and Depression Score
5. Edmonton Symptom Assessment (palliative care)
6. FLACC or CRIES score for neonates
7. COMFORT pain scales. Observation of neonates (4)

D. **Give 4 methods of assessing acute pain** (4 marks)

1. History and examination/observation
2. Visual Analogue Score
3. Numerical Rating Score
4. Verbal rating scale
5. Faces Pain Scale (4)

E. Give 4 problems with these assessment tools? (4 marks)

1. Unidimensional
2. Snapshot in time
3. Pain at rest or when moving may be very different
4. Patient may not understand the test (age, language, cognition, deafness)
5. Subjective measure only
6. Pain memory not always accurate (e.g. during last 24 hours or last 7 days) (4)

Total 20 marks

Further reading

H Breivik, PC Borchgrevink, SM Allen, et al; Assessment of pain, *BJA: British Journal of Anaesthesia*, Volume 101, Issue 1, 1 July 2008, Pages 17–24.

S Callin, MI Bennett; Assessment of neuropathic pain, *Continuing Education in Anaesthesia Critical Care & Pain*, Volume 8, Issue 6, 1 December 2008, Pages 210–213.

IASP Definition of Pain, *Pain*, Volume 6, 1979, Page 250.

Question 4

A 21-year-old man is listed for dental extractions (UR8, LR8, UL8, LL8) as a day case. His only medical history is vWD type 1 associated with easy bruising.

A. Define vWD (2 marks)

1. vWD is an inherited disorder
2. It is caused by missing or defective von Willebrand factor (VWF)
3. It results in a bleeding tendency (2)

B. What is the specific role of von Willebrand's Factor? (1 mark)

1. Von Willebrand's Factor's primary function is binding to factor VIII
2. It is important in platelet adhesion at wound sites (1)

C. Indicate the likely findings on blood testing. In the boxes enter raised [↑], decreased [↓], or normal [↔] for each parameter (1 mark awarded for each correct pair of answers to a maximum of 3 marks)

	Platelet count	Bleeding time	APTT	PT	Fibrinogen	Factor VIII level
Von Willebrand's disease	↔	↑	↑	↔	↔	↓

Note: 1 mark for each consecutive pair correct (3)

D. The patient attends the preoperative assessment clinic. What logistics, investigations, and specific therapies should be considered prior to presenting for surgery?

Logistics (2 marks)	1. Discussion with haematologist 2. Ensure 1st on list/morning list 3. Ensure overnight admission bed availability if needed
Investigations (2 marks)	1. Full blood count and coagulation assay 2. Blood group and antibody screen 3. Factor VIII/vWF levels prior to surgery (to ensure 50–100% of normal levels)
Specific therapies (2 marks)	1. Plan desmopressin (DDAVP) prophylactically 90 mins before surgery (assuming positive responder) 2. Recombinant factor VIII or cryoprecipitate if non-responder to DDAVP

(6)

E. The patient presents on day of surgery. Describe the advantages and disadvantages of endotracheal intubation via the nasal route in this patient (3 marks)?

	Advantage (1 mark)	Disadvantages (2 marks)
Nasal intubation	1. Improved surgical access for bilateral wisdom teeth extractions	1. Risk of nosebleed in patient with prolonged bleeding time 2. Inability to pass through obstructed nose 3. Longer and narrower tube with increased airway pressure requirement or potential to kink

(3)

F. How can intra- and postoperative bleeding be minimized during this case? (5 marks)

1. Avoid NSAIDs
2. Avoidance of hypertension and tachycardia
3. DDAVP administration
4. Aim factor VIII levels >50% of normal
5. Tranexamic acid
6. Use of local anaesthesia with adrenaline
7. Meticulous surgical technique and limiting the duration of procedure
8. Use of local pressure–biting on a swab
9. Nasal packing if nose bleeds
10. Head-up tilt, avoidance of venous congestion   (5)

Total 20 marks

Further reading

UJ Shah, M Narayanan, JG Smith; Anaesthetic considerations in patients with inherited disorders of coagulation, *Continuing Education in Anaesthesia Critical Care & Pain*, Volume 15, Issue 1, 2015, Pages 26–31.

Question 5

A. What factors must you take into account for consent to be considered 'informed'? (5 marks)

1. Patient must have capacity
2. Patient must be able to receive and understand the information provided
3. Patient must be free to make a balanced decision free from coercion
4. Information must be rational and stand up to logical analysis
5. Doctor must mention significant hazards (as to the importance the patient would place upon them) even if rare and to discuss alternatives including no treatment
6. Patient can withdraw consent at any time—assuming retains capacity

Note: any 5 answers for marks   (5)

B. Name 2 acts of parliament which legislate for capacity to consent in the UK (2 marks)

1. The Mental Health Act 1985 England and Wales
2. The Mental Capacity Act 2005 England and Wales
3. Adults with Incapacity Act 2000 Scotland
4. The Mental capacity Act 2016 Northern Ireland

Note: Any 2 of the aforementioned options required for marks   (2)

C. **What change to the consent process evolved from the Montgomery versus Lanarkshire Health Board judgement handed down March 2015?** (3 marks)

1. Informed consent addresses risks
2. Previously, explain risks as a reasonable doctor would consider appropriate (Hunter vs. Hanley 1955 and Bolam 1957)
3. Now must discuss all material risks that any reasonable patient would wish to know or would attach significance to, and also where the doctor believes this to be the case   (3)

D. **What difficulties are there in explaining risks to a patient?** (4 marks)

1. Population statistics do not apply to individuals. If a rare complication occurs, the rate is 100% in the patient affected despite the risk being extremely low on a population basis.
2. Patients find it difficult to fully comprehend what is meant by subjective terms such as 'very common' or 'very rare'. The Royal College of Anaesthetists (RCoA) suggests we link numbers with pictures or diagrams (infographics) to tell patients that:
   - Very common is 1 in 10, equivalent to someone in their family being affected
   - Common is 1 in 100 being someone in your street, and
   - Uncommon meaning 1 in 1,000 or someone in a village
   - Rare to be 1 in 10,000, and
   - Very rare to be 1 in 100,000, equivalent to one person in a large town.
3. Patients do not expect to be affected by low risk events
4. Different patients may feel differently about the same level of risk (risk takers, risk averse, or if they know someone who was affected by the adverse event)   (4)

E. **What is a Caldicott Guardian?** (2 marks)

1. A Caldicott Guardian is a person responsible for protecting the confidentiality of peoples' health and care information,
2. They make sure information is governed properly.   (2)

F. **What are the 4 principles of ethical decision-making that must be considered in clinical practice?** (4 marks)

MORAL Balance

   M: Make sure of the facts

   OR: identify Outcomes of Relevance …

   A: for the Agents involved

   L: populate then Level out the arguments with

   BALANCE: identify conflict and congruent points and their place in the 4 ethical principles.

Reprinted from *BJA Education*, 19(3), D. J.R. Harvey and D. Gardiner, 'MORAL balance' decision-making in critical care. 68–73. Copyright © 2019, with permission from Elsevier Ltd., British Journal of Anaesthetists and The Royal College of Anaesthetists. doi: 10.1016/j.bjae.2018.11.006

          (4)

Note: only 1 mark available for 'M' or 'O'

Total 20 marks

Further reading

Disability Matters https://www.disabilitymatters.org.uk

GMC Rules on Consent https://www.gmc-uk.org/ethical-guidance/ethical-guidance-for-doctors/consent

DJR Harvey, D Gardiner; MORAL balance decision-making in critical care, *BJA Education*, Volume 19, Issue 3, 2019, Page 68e73.

T Orr, R Baruah; Consent in anaesthesia, critical care and pain medicine. *BJA Education*, Volume 18, Issue 5, 2018, Pages 135–139.

Royal College of Anaesthetists (RCoA); Consent and ethics for children and young people https://www.rcoa.ac.uk/documents/consent-ethics-children-young-people/consent

Royal College of Anaesthetists (RCoA); New rules on consent 2015 https://www.rcoa.ac.uk/sites/default/files/documents/2009-11/Guideline_ consent_for_anaesthesia_2007_final%20%281%29%20to%20be%20uploaded.pdf

UK Caldicott Guardian Council https://www.gov.uk/government/groups/uk-caldicott-guardian-council

Question 6

A 73-year-old man presents with a gangrenous left foot and requires an urgent below-knee amputation. He is known to have peripheral vascular disease, previous CVA, COPD, and stable angina. His current medication includes clopidogrel, ramipril, simvastatin, isosorbide mononitrate. He also takes zomorph 30mg b.d. with sevredol 5mg for breakthrough pain and regular paracetamol for ischaemic limb pain.

A. **List 3 risk factors for the development of phantom limb pain postoperatively** (3 marks)

1. Severe preoperative pain
2. Bilateral amputations
3. Increasing age
4. Stump pain
5. Repeated limb surgeries (3)

B. **Outline your management of this patient to treat acute pain and attenuate the likelihood of developing chronic pain following amputation, using the subheadings that follow next.**

Preoperative (3 marks)
1. Optimize pain control preoperatively to achieve good pain relief
2. Maintain usual pain medications
3. Increase/bolus opioids if necessary
4. Pregabalin/gabapentin premedication if not already taking
5. Consider salmon calcitonin (100 units/day subcutaneously for 5–7 days) (3)

Intraoperative (3 marks)
1. Continuous sciatic nerve block with catheter—popliteal.
2. Ketamine as bolus +/− infusion
3. Consider clonidine
4. (Epidural and spinal contraindicated due to clopidogrel) (3)

Postoperative (5 marks)

1. Continue sciatic nerve block for >72 hours most important
2. Regular opioid and paracetamol plus breakthrough prescribed. Consider PCA
3. Continue pregabalin/gabapentin
4. Low dose ketamine infusion if pain control poor
5. Ensure followed up daily by the acute pain team to address any issues early
6. Physiotherapy and early mobilization

Note: Must have sciatic block for full marks (5)

C. Outline the correct process during 'Stop Before You Block' (2 marks)

1. WHO checklist performed
2. Visualize surgical arrow indicating site of surgery
3. Ask the patient to confirm the side of surgery (if conscious)
4. Double check the consent form for operative site (if patient unconscious) (2)

D. Give the 2 main branches of the sciatic nerve. Describe the motor response elicited by stimulation of each nerve (4 marks)

Nerve (2 marks)	Motor response (2 marks)
1. Tibial nerve	1. Plantarflexion of the foot
2. Common peroneal nerve	2. Eversion and dorsiflexion of the foot

(4)

Total 20 marks

Further reading

MJE Neil; Pain after amputation, *BJA Education*, Volume 16, Issue 3, March 2016, Pages 107–112.

Question 7

A 68-year-old man is known to have aortic stenosis.

A. List 3 cardinal symptoms of worsening aortic stenosis? (3 marks)

1. Angina
2. Syncope
3. Breathlessness (3)

B. What are the 3 most common causes of aortic stenosis? (3 marks)

   1. Degenerative calcific stenosis
   2. Congenital bicuspid aortic valve
   3. Rheumatic fever as a child   (3)

C. Describe the pathophysiology of worsening aortic stenosis (3 marks)

   1. Left ventricular hypertrophy in response to outflow obstruction
   2. Reduced compliance of the hypertrophied ventricle causes diastolic dysfunction
   3. Left ventricle (LV) dilation occurs late
   4. End stage is congestive cardiac failure   (3)

D. He attends preoperative assessment during workup for consideration of a valve intervention.
   What are the expected abnormal findings in aortic stenosis? (4 marks)

Clinical examination signs (2 marks)	1. Slow rising pulse 2. Low volume pulse 3. Systolic murmur at 2nd Right intercostal space 4. Radiation to carotid (bruit)
ECG findings (1 mark)	1. Left ventricular hypertrophy 2. T-wave inversion/ST segment depression 3. AV blocks
CXR findings (1 mark)	1. Valve calcification 2. Left ventricular failure signs—appear late

                                                                               (4)

E. An updated echocardiogram is requested as part of the preoperative assessment.

   Describe 3 specific measurements on echocardiography indicating severe aortic stenosis?
   (3 marks)

   1. Aortic jet velocity >4m/s
   2. Peak gradient >65mmHg
   3. Mean gradient >40mmHg
   4. Valve area <1cm^2
   5. Valve area indexed <0.6cm^{2}m^{-2}BSA
   6. Consequences of severe aortic stenosis (e.g. poor LV function/dilatation)   (3)

F. List 3 potential valve interventions for severe symptomatic aortic stenosis? (1 mark)

1. Aortic valve replacement (AVR)
2. Transcatheter aortic valve implantation (TAVI)
3. Balloon valvuloplasty

Note: Need all 3 for 1 mark   (1)

G. You plan to anaesthetise the patient for valve intervention.

What are the cardiovascular goals specific to aortic stenosis for this patient? (3 marks)
1. Ideal heart rate 60–80 beats per minute (tachycardia is poorly tolerated as inadequate diastolic time for coronary filling)
2. Maintenance of sinus rhythm (AF poorly tolerated in AS)
3. Maintain adequate systemic pressure
4. Maintain contractility
5. Optimize preload for a non-compliant ventricle   (3)

Total 20 marks

Further reading

J Brown, NJ Morgan-Hughes; Aortic stenosis and non-cardiac surgery, *Continuing Education in Anaesthesia Critical Care & Pain*, Volume 5, Issue 1, 2005, Pages 1–4.

M Chacko, L Weinberg; Aortic valve stenosis: perioperative anaesthetic implications of surgical replacement and minimally invasive interventions, *Continuing Education in Anaesthesia Critical Care & Pain*, Volume 12, Issue 6, 2012, Pages 295–301.

Question 8

A 59-year-old man is scheduled for an elective lumbar discectomy. At the preassessment clinic the nurse is concerned he may have OSA.

A. Complete the STOP-BANG scoring tool for OSA (8 marks)

S (1 mark)	Do you snore loudly?
T (1 mark)	Do you feel tired during the day most days?
O (1 mark)	Has anyone observed you stop breathing during your sleep?
P (1 mark)	History of high blood pressure?
B (1 mark)	BMI >35
A (1 mark)	Age over 50

N (1 mark)	Neck circumference > 40cm
G (1 mark)	Male gender

(8)

Note: High risk for OSA if > 3 criteria.

B. **What are the endocrine** (3 marks) **and cardiovascular** (3 marks) **consequences of OSA?**

Endocrine (3 marks)

1. Impaired glucose tolerance
2. Dyslipidaemia
3. Testicular/ovarian dysfunction
4. Altered hypothalamic–pituitary–adrenal response with increased adrenocorticotropic hormone (ACTH) and cortisol levels

(3)

Cardiovascular (3 marks)

1. Systemic hypertension
2. Pulmonary hypertension
3. Right ventricular failure/ heart failure
4. Dysrhythmias
5. Increased risk of myocardial infarction and stroke
6. Pickwickian syndrome

(3)

C. **This patient is investigated and diagnosed with OSA. You intend to use high-flow nasal oxygen therapy for preoxygenation and postoperatively. What are the specifics of high-flow nasal oxygen therapy which confer physiological advantage?** (6 marks)

High gas flow up to 60L/min

1. Gives FiO_2 close to 1.0
2. Causes CO_2 washout
3. Reduction in the dead space
4. Increases the oxygen reservoir thereby improving oxygenation.

Warmed humidified gas

1. Reduces heat and moisture loss form the airway
2. Improves secretion clearance
3. Decreases atelectasis.

Delivers PEEP

1. increases end expiratory lung volume and alveolar recruitment
2. reduces the work of breathing

Note: Must have at least one answer from each of the 3 categories for full marks. (6)

Total 20 marks

Further reading

N Ashraf-Kashani, R Kumar; High-flow nasal oxygen therapy, *BJA Education*, Volume 17, Issue 2, February 2017, Pages 57–62.

G Martinez, P Faber; Obstructive sleep apnoea, *Continuing Education in Anaesthesia Critical Care & Pain*, Volume 11, Issue 1, February 2011, Pages 5–8.

Question 9

A 90-year-old woman with a fractured neck of femur is scheduled for operative fixation with a dynamic hip screw. She weighs 45kg. She has AF and takes digoxin 125μg, warfarin 5mg, and furosemide 20mg daily. Her blood pressure is 150/90mmHg and heart rate is 80 beats per minute.

A. **Define frailty syndrome** (1 mark)

In-built physiological reserves gradually decline with age leaving weakness of the body and mind, prone to sudden changes in health triggered by seemingly small events, including minor infections or a change in medication or environment. (1)

Note: In medicine, frailty defines the group of older people who are at highest risk of adverse outcomes such as falls, disability, admission to hospital, or the need for long-term care.

B. From the information in the question, what underlying comorbidities may have caused her fall? Complete the table with at least one cause in each category (5 marks–one mark per column)

CVS	CNS	Metabolic	Global changes with age	Infection
Arrythmia	$transient ischaemic attack (TIA)/CVA (ischaemic/embolic)	Hyponatraemia	Reduced muscle mass Reduced strength	
Postural hypotension	Acute confusional state	Hypokalaemia	Reduced proprioception	
		Dehydration	Reduced eyesight	

Causes below may occur too but are not specifically reasons expected from the history in this case

Acute coronary syndrome	Parkinson's	Hypoglycaemia		Chest and urinary sources common
Valvular heart disease				

(5)

Note: 90% such falls are simple trips and falls whereas only 10% are attributable to a comorbidity

C. Complete the table to show the advantages of general versus advantages of regional anaesthesia in this patient?

	Advantages
General anaesthesia (3 marks)	1. Airway and breathing secured and controlled in a sick patient
	2. Potentially more cardiostable through induction and maintenance
	3. Reduced need for compliance from the patient
	4. Positioning facilitated and tolerated throughout

Regional anaesthesia (3 marks)	1. Reduced risk of postoperative cognitive dysfunction (POCD) including delirium.
	2. Good postoperative analgesia with minimal systemic polypharmacy
	3. No requirement to instrument the airway or manage artificial ventilation
	4. Decreased risk of venous thromboembolism (VTE) events

Note: 1 mark given for each correct statement to a maximum of 3 in each section. Marks not given for general comparisons of these techniques. (6)

D. **How would you manage her anticoagulation perioperatively** (3 marks)

1. Stop warfarin
2. Check INR<1.5
3. May require IV vitamin K and/or prothrombin complex concentrate (Octaplex)
4. Commence unfractionated low molecular weight heparin for venous thromboembolic prophylaxis
5. No role for aspirin as risk of bleeding outweighs the potential benefit in this population. (3)

E. **What formal scoring system could you use to estimate her risk of morbidity and mortality?** (1 mark)

1. Nottingham Hip Fracture Score
2. SORT: surgical outcome risk tool
3. P-POSSUM: Physiological and operative severity score for the enumeration of mortality and morbidity (Portsmouth predictor equation). (1)

F. **List 4 of the variables which increase the risk of mortality at 30 days in the frail population** (4 marks)

1. Low Hb <100g/L
2. Mini Mental Test Score (MMTS)
3. Number of comorbidities
4. Living in an institution
5. Malignancy
6. Age
7. Sex (4)

Total 20 marks

Further reading

CM O'Donnell, L McLoughlin, CC Patterson, et al.; Perioperative outcomes in the context of mode of anaesthesia for patients undergoing hip fracture surgery: systematic review and meta-analysis, *British Journal of Anaesthesia*, Volume 120, Issue 1, Pages 37–50.

IK Moppett, M Parker, R Griffiths, T Bowers, SM White, CG Moran; Nottingham Hip Fracture Score: longitudinal and multi-centre assessment, *BJA: British Journal of Anaesthesia*, Volume 109, Issue 4, October 2012, Pages 546–550.

Royal College Physicians London; *National Hip Fracture Database Annual Report 2018*, http://bit.ly/2DjbA4F

UJ Shah, M Narayanan, J Graham Smith; Anaesthetic considerations in patients with inherited disorders of coagulation, *Continuing Education in Anaesthesia Critical Care & Pain*, Volume 15, Issue 1, February 2015, Pages 26–31.

Note: For completeness the CHA_2DS_2-VASc

score stratifies the annual risk of a thromboembolic stroke in patients with AF.

Score 0 is 2%, up to score 6 is 18.2%. Score >3 anticoagulate

CHA_2DS_2-VASc

C—congestive cardiac failure

H—hypertension160/90

A—age over 75 years

D—presence of diabetes mellitus

S—stroke or TIA previously

V   Vascular disease (e.g. peripheral artery disease, myocardial infarction, aortic plaque)

A   Age 65–74 years

Sc   Sex category (i.e. female sex)

Question 10

In the preassessment clinic, a 62-year-old patient requires hysterectomy for endometrial cancer. She has hypertension, depression, back pain, and fibromyalgia. Her BMI is 45.

She takes lisinopril, sertraline, co-codamol (30/500) 8 tablets per day, oxycodone 40mg b.d., and shortec 10mg for breakthrough pain, which she usually requires twice per day. The gynaecologists do not wish to postpone her operation.

A. Describe the main perioperative pain management issue in this patient (1 mark)

She is on a significant dose of opioids preoperatively and will be opioid tolerant and physiologically dependent   (1)

B. How much OME does she take in 24 hours? (2 marks)

1. Co-codamol: 240 mg codeine = 24mg morphine.
2. Oxycodone 80mg = 160 mg morphine
3. Shortec 20mg = 40 mg morphine

Note: Total 224 mg (accept 200mg) (2)

C. What specific measures would you take to reduce the impact this has perioperatively? (4 marks).

1. Pre-op discussion regarding benefits of slow tapered reduction prior to operation
2. Continue her usual opioid regime as far as possible throughout her admission
3. Use regional analgesic techniques as far as possible
4. Consider changing to a sole preparation of oral/IV morphine only
5. Ask for help and advice from acute pain team and pharmacist (4)

D. Outline your plan for perioperative analgesia (6 marks)

Preoperative period

1. Consider preoperative dose of gabapentinoids
2. Continue usual medication as long as possible (1)

Intraoperative measures

1. Regional anaesthesia plus GA
2. Option of intrathecal local anaesthesia plus opioid, or an epidural bolus
3. Nitrous oxide
4. Consider local anaesthetic infiltration to wound by surgeon
5. Consider lidocaine infusion (3)

Postoperatively

1. Epidural infusion
2. Consider wound catheter with local anaesthetic
3. Adjuncts: paracetamol 1g regularly, max 4g/ day (caution: co-codamol)
4. Consider short course (48 hours) NSAIDS
5. PCA morphine (2)

Note: no additional mark for stating epidural twice

E. You are called to review her in recovery as she reports severe pain. She is using a standard PCA regime of 1 mg morphine bolus with a 5-minute lockout. Give 2 ways you can increase the efficacy of this PCA (2 marks)

1. Increase the bolus dose
2. Add a background infusion
3. Consider an opioid switch to oxycodone or fentanyl due to incomplete cross tolerance (2)

F. What other analgesics might you consider at this stage? (1 mark)

Low dose ketamine infusion (1)

G. What are your instructions on discharge from recovery? (2 marks)

1. Observe in HDU
2. Monitor for opioid toxicity, respiratory depression, and drowsiness
3. Monitor oxygen saturation
4. Continue PCA until can restarting of usual oral medications (2)

H. What other classes of drugs might you prescribe for the postoperative period? (2 marks)

1. Antiemetic (nausea)
2. Stat dose of naloxone IM/IV as required for itch
3. Antihistamine/ondansetron (itch)
4. Laxatives (constipation) (2)

Total 20 marks

Further reading

GK Simpson, M Jackson; Perioperative management of opioid-tolerant patients, *BJA Education*, Volume 17, Issue 4, April 2017, Pages 124–128.

Question 11

You have been called to the ED to review a 24-year-old man with a significant traumatic brain injury, following an assault. He has no other injuries.

A. What would be the indications to intubate and ventilate this patient? (8 marks)

1. Glasgow Coma score <8
2. Significantly deteriorating conscious level even if >8 (fall of > 2 points)
3. Loss of protective airway reflexes or high risk of aspiration
4. Evidence of ventilatory insufficiency despite high-flow oxygen (e.g. low PaO_2 or high $PaCO_2$)
5. Spontaneous hyperventilation with a $PaCO_2$ <4kPa
6. Irregular respiration
7. Seizures
8. Unstable facial fractures
9. Bleeding into the mouth
10. For transfer to a tertiary neurosurgical centre (8)

B. You intubate and ventilate the patient successfully with cervical spine stabilization and prepare for transfer. Outline your management to prevent secondary brain injury (6 marks)

1. Secure ET tube carefully to avoid obstruction to cerebral venous drainage
2. Position with a 30-degree head-up tilt
3. Ensure adequate sedation, analgesia, and muscle relaxation
4. Maintain a PaO_2 >13kPa
5. Maintain a $PaCO_2$ of 4–4.5kPA
6. Maintain a mean arterial blood pressure (MABP) >80mmHg with fluids +/- vasopressors
7. Check blood glucose level and maintain normoglycaemia
8. Urinary catheterization (urinary retention can lead to raised ICP)
9. Maintain core temperature 35–37°C/avoid hyperthermia

Note: Must have ventilatory targets and MABP target to get all marks   (6)

C. What are the 2 recommended values to target to prevent secondary brain injury? (2 marks)

Intracranial pressure (1 mark)	≤20–25mmHg (≤ 35cm H_2O)
Cerebral perfusion pressure (1 mark)	≥60mmHg (≥ 80cm H_2O)

(2)

D. The patient is transferred safely to the tertiary neurosurgical centre where they find his intracranial pressure is raised, despite your management.

What further options are there to reduce intracranial pressure? (4 marks)

1. Hyperventilation to a $PaCO_2$ 4–4.5kPA
2. Use of osmotic diuretic such as mannitol
3. Hypothermia
4. Intravenous barbiturates
5. Surgical interventions   (4)

Total 20 marks

Further reading

The Association of Anaesthetists of Great Britain and Ireland; *Recommendations for the Safe Transfer of Patients with Brain Injury*, 2006 https://anaesthetists.org/Home/News-opinion/News/Updated-guidelines-for-safe-transfer-of-patients-with-a-brain-injury

J Dinsmore, Traumatic brain injury: an evidence-based review of management, *Continuing Education in Anaesthesia Critical Care & Pain*, Volume 13, Issue 6, December 2013, Pages 189–195.

Question 12

You are asked to see a 24-year-old woman on the postnatal ward who is 36 hours following a spontaneous vaginal delivery. She had an epidural in labour. She is now complaining of severe headache. You suspect a PDPH.

A. List 6 other possible causes of a headache in this patient (6 marks)

1. Tension headache
2. Migraine
3. Dehydration
4. Pre-eclampsia/hypertension
5. Subarachnoid haemorrhage
6. Cavernous sinus thrombosis
7. Central nervous system infection (e.g. meningitis)
8. Space occupying lesion
9. Caffeine withdrawal headache (6)

B. Describe the pathophysiology of headache in PDPH (3 marks)

1. Cerebrospinal fluid (CSF) leaks through the dural puncture
2. Intracranial hypotension results
3. The postural headache is thought to be triggered by vascular distension/dilation that occurs on standing
4. An increased hydrostatic gradient on standing forces yet more CSF leakage
5. Adenosine receptors may be activated to compensate for the sudden loss of intracranial volume (3)

C. List 5 classical symptoms of PDPH (5 marks)

1. Fronto-occipital location of pain
2. Postural component (worse on standing)
3. Worse with coughing/straining
4. Neck stiffness
5. Nausea/vomiting
6. Photophobia
7. Auditory symptoms—hearing loss, tinnitus, hyperacusis (5)

D. The patient is also complaining of double vision. Describe a likely cause and specific findings on neurological examination (2 marks)

1. In severe cases a 6th cranial nerve palsy (abducens) may occur
2. Clinical features are failure of lateral movement of the eye on the affected side (2)

E. **List 3 options for management of postdural puncture headache symptoms** (3 marks)

1. Simple analgesics
2. Caffeine
3. Hydration
4. 5HT-agonists
5. Epidural blood patch (3)

Note: There is poor evidence for most of the traditional conservative measures of caffeine, hydration, and multiple other pharmacological agents including these points, yet they continue to be prescribed.

F. **What factor has the most impact in reducing the incidence of PDPH associated with lumbar epidural?** (1 mark)

1. Highly experienced operator
2. Choice of higher gauge (smaller) regional needles for a neuraxial technique, e.g. 18 gauge Tuohy needle preferred over a 16 gauge (1)

Total 20 marks

Further reading

A Sabharwal, GM Stocks; Postpartum headache: diagnosis and management, *Continuing Education in Anaesthesia Critical Care & Pain*, Volume 11, Issue 5, 1 October 2011, Pages 181–185.

Exam 3 Questions

Exam 3 contains 12 selected Constructed Response Questions (CRQs) balanced across the intermediate curriculum, reflecting the Final Fellowship of the Royal College of Anaesthetists (FRCA) exam. We recommend attempting these questions under exam conditions. **Please limit/contain your answer to/within the dotted lines given for each question.**

Question 1

A 56-year-old man attends for trans-sphenoid resection of hypophyseal tumour. He has a long history of headaches and blurred vision. The diagnosis is of benign pituitary adenoma and he has clinical features of acromegaly.

A. What pathophysiology causes acromegaly? (1 mark)

....

B. Which other hormones are secreted from the pituitary gland? (2 marks)

Location in pituitary	Hormones secreted
Anterior lobe (1 mark)	1. .... 2. .... 3. .... 4. ....
Posterior lobe (1 mark)	1. .... 2. ....

C. What are the patient-specific features of acromegaly which are relevant to anaesthesia? (4 marks)

1. ....

2. ....

3. ....

4. ....

D. What are the special considerations within the anaesthetic management of this patient for trans-sphenoidal hypophysectomy that you would consider in your preoperative assessment? (5 marks)

E. The surgeon asks you to facilitate a bloodless field. What can you do to help? (2 marks)

F. You plan to awaken and extubate the patient immediately at the end of the procedure. What homeostatic variables must be achieved to facilitate this? (3 marks)

G. You plan to place the patient in high dependency unit (HDU) postoperatively. What specific management should be instituted for this patient as an adjunct to standard HDU care? (3 marks)

....

....

....

Total 20 marks

Question 2

A 39-year-old female is listed for deep inferior epigastric perforator (DIEP) breast reconstruction. Her only medical history is breast cancer.

A. Outline the 2 main categories of autologous flap blood supply used in plastic surgery (2 marks)

1. ....

2. ....

B. What are the physical determinants of blood flow through a flap? (4 marks). State their relationship to one another (1 mark)

1. ....

2. ....

3. ....

4. ....

....

....

C. What non-standard monitoring is considered appropriate for this procedure? (3 marks)

1. ....

2. ....

3. ....

D. What are the intraoperative physiological goals targeted to improve the chances of flap survival? (6 marks)

1. ....

2. ....

3. ....

4. ....

5. ....

6. ....

E. In recovery there are concerns regarding the perfusion of the flap.

How can flap perfusion be assessed clinically at the bedside in the postoperative period? (4 marks)

1. ....

2. ....

3. ....

4. ....

Total 20 marks

Question 3

A 67-year-old man is scheduled for laryngoscopy and biopsy for suspected carcinoma. The surgeon has requested a tubeless field so you have therefore decided to use total intravenous anaesthesia (TIVA).

A. List 5 other specific indications for TIVA (5 marks)

1. ....

2. ....

3. ....

4. ....

5. ....

B. You are using a target-controlled infusion (TCI) of propofol.

Outline the key components of a TCI device (4 marks)

....

....

....

....

....

....

C. List 2 pharmacokinetic adult models used for propofol (2 marks)

1. ....

2. ....

D. Describe the three-compartment pharmacokinetic model for propofol (5 marks)

E. Describe how a TCI device ensures a steady state concentration of a drug (4 marks)

Total 20 marks

Question 4

You and your consultant are about to perform brainstem death testing on a 64-year-old woman in the intensive care unit (ICU).

A. List 4 'red flags' when diagnostic caution is advised for brainstem death testing? (4 marks)

1. ....

2. ....

3. ....

4. ....

B. Describe how you would perform the apnoea test as part of the brainstem death testing? (6 marks)

....

....

....

....

....

....

....

....

....

C. You have completed both sets of brainstem death tests, confirmed death by neurological criteria and spoken with the family. The patient is going to proceed to organ donation. She currently has an arterial blood pressure of 84/39mmHg and a central venous pressure (CVP) of 3cmH$_2$O.

Outline your cardiovascular targets for this patient to maximize donor potential (3 marks)

Heart rate range (bpm) (1 mark)	
Mean arterial pressure range (mmHg) (1 mark)	
CVP range (mmHg) (1 mark)	

D. How would you achieve these cardiovascular targets? (2 marks)

....

....

E. This patient has a urine output of over 400ml/hour.

What biochemical features would confirm the diagnosis of diabetes insipidus? (2 marks)

....

....

F. Outline your management of the main endocrine abnormalities that occur after brainstem death (3 marks)

....

....

Total 20 marks

Question 5

A 32-year-old woman attends for pelvic laparoscopy. She weighs 70kg and her body mass index (BMI) is 35. Her medical history is severe reflux. She had generalized muscular ache following administration of suxamethonium during a previous anaesthetic. Her medication is omeprazole 20mg bd and the oral contraceptive pill. You decide to use rocuronium to facilitate intubation.

A. Give 5 other advantages of using rocuronium instead of suxamethonium for a rapid sequence induction (5 marks)

1. ....

2. ....

3. ....

4. ....

5. ....

B. What dose of rocuronium would you use for a rapid sequence induction in this patient? (1 mark)

....

C. Describe the pharmacodynamic principle which accounts for rocuronium's more rapid onset of action when compared to vecuronium? (2 marks)

1. ....

....

2. ....

....

D. Give 2 processes by which the effects of rocuronium can be terminated at the end of the procedure (2 marks)

1. ....

2. ....

E. Explain the pharmacology of each method (4 marks)

Process 1

....

....

....

....

....

....

....

Process 2

F. What dose of sugammadex would you precalculate for immediate reversal of rocuronium in the event of a failed intubation in this patient? (1 mark)

G. 30 minutes later in the recovery room the patient is hypotensive and is to return to theatre with suspected intra-abdominal bleeding.

Give 3 drug options available to facilitate laryngoscopy conditions during repeat intubation (3 marks)

1.

2.

3.

H. What postoperative advice would you give to this patient regarding their administration of sugammadex? (2 marks)

Total 20 marks

Question 6

A company representative attends your department one lunchtime to showcase their new ultrasound machine.

A. Give 4 examples each of diagnostic and therapeutic uses of ultrasound in anaesthetic and critical care practice? (8 marks)

Diagnostic

1. ....

2. ....

3. ....

4. ....

Therapeutic

1. ....

2. ....

3. ....

4. ....

B. What is the Doppler effect? (2 marks)

....

....

C. Give 2 applications of the Doppler effect used in echocardiography? (2 marks)

1. ....

2. ....

D. What information can echocardiography provide in a haemodynamically unstable patient?
(8 marks)

1. ....

2. ....

3. ....

4. ....

5. ....

6. ....

7. ....

8. ....

Total 20 marks

Question 7

A 59-year-old woman has presented with gradual onset leg weakness and now has difficulty walking. She is normally fit and well but had a self-limiting episode of gastroenteritis 3 weeks ago. She takes no regular medication.

A. List the classic clinical features of Guillain-Barré syndrome (GBS) (5 marks)

....

....

....

....

....

B. What specific investigations, with their findings, would support a diagnosis of GBS? (6 marks)

C. The patient is admitted to HDU and she is investigated for suspected GBS. However, over the last 48 hours she develops symmetrical arm weakness as well. Today she is struggling to cough and swallow and her respiratory rate has increased to 32 breaths/min. Her PaO_2 is 8.9kPA on 70% oxygen.

You decide she needs ventilatory support.

What specific modifications would you make to your induction and intubating technique for this patient? (2 marks)

D. You intubate without incident. She is now ventilated and fully monitored, with an arterial and central line, in ICU.

Outline your ongoing specific (2 marks) and supportive management (5 marks) for this patient.

Specific

1. ....

2. ....

Supportive

1. ....

2. ....

3. ....

4. ....

5. ....

Total 20 marks

Question 8

You receive a trauma call to the ED. A 22-year old man was the driver of a car involved in a high-speed road traffic collision. He has multiple injuries.

A. You suspect an immediate life-threatening thoracic injury. List 5 treatable causes of this found on primary survey (5 marks)

1. ....

2. ....

3. ....

4. ....

5. ....

B. What immediate diagnostic imaging is appropriate for diagnosing chest trauma? (2 marks)

1. ....

2. ....

C. Primary survey is now complete. The patient is breathing spontaneously but not moving his arms or legs. A C5 cervical spine injury is suspected.

What are the clinical features on examination of an acute C5 cervical spine injury? (5 marks)

1. ....

2. ....

3. ....

4. ....

5. ....

D. Describe the specific modifications to airway management during a rapid sequence induction of anaesthesia for this patient (4 marks)

1. ....

2. ....

3. ....

4. ....

E. One month later the patient is transferred to a spinal injuries unit.

Briefly describe these clinical syndromes resulting from spinal cord injury (4 marks)

Syndrome	Description
Anterior spinal artery syndrome (2 marks)	
Brown-Séquard syndrome (2 marks)	

Total 20 marks

Question 9

You are to anaesthetise a 78-year-old woman for an elective right total hip replacement. She weighs 51kg and has a past medical history including stable angina, hypertension, chronic obstructive pulmonary disease (COPD), and peripheral vascular disease. You plan a spinal anaesthetic with a target-controlled infusion of propofol (TCI) for deep sedation.

A. Define inadvertent perioperative hypothermia (IPH)? (1 mark)

B. This patient's temperature on arrival in the theatre suite is 35.4°C.

List 5 risk factors for the development of IPH in the general patient? (5 marks)

1. ....

2. ....

3. ....

4. ....

5. ....

C. Describe in detail 4 major consequences and the associated pathophysiology of IPH that may impact the morbidity and mortality of patients (8 marks)

Major consequence of IPH (4 marks)	Pathophysiology (4 marks)

D. Outline your management of this patient's temperature before and during surgery (6 marks)

....

....

....

....

....

....

Total 20 marks

Question 10

A 32-year-old woman, Para 2 + 0 is having a caesarean section under spinal anaesthesia.

The baby and placenta have been delivered successfully but there is ongoing bleeding of approximately 800mls so far.

A. List the 4 main causes of primary postpartum haemorrhage (PPH) (4 marks)

1. ....

2. ....

3. ....

4. ....

B. Complete the table of drugs used to treat uterine atony as directed. Give their doses and routes of administration. List their mechanisms of action and common side effects (12 marks)

Drug	Doses and routes of administration	Mechanism of action	Side effects
Oxytocin (3 marks)			
Ergometrine (3 marks)			
Carboprost (3 marks)			
Misoprostol (3 marks)			

C. Despite the appropriate administration of uterotonics over the last 20 minutes and administration of 2L of crystalloid, the bleeding is ongoing with blood loss now at 1.5L.

Outline the next steps in your management of this patient (4 marks)

....

....

....

....

....

....

Total 20 marks

Question 11

A 6-year-old girl requires elective tonsillectomy. She has no significant medical history.

A. Briefly describe 2 indications for paediatric tonsillectomy (2 marks)

1. ....

2. ....

B. Regarding the choice of airway technique for this case, what are the advantages of each below? (6 marks)

	Laryngeal mask airway (LMA) (3 marks)	Tracheal Intubation (3 marks)
Advantages	1.	1. ....
	2.	2. ....
	3.	3. ....

C. She re-presents as an emergency 12 hours postoperatively with bleeding from the tonsillar bed. The ears, nose and throat (ENT) surgeon wishes to expedite her return to theatre.

List 4 clinical challenges pertaining to this case (4 marks)

1. ....

2. ....

3. ....

4. ....

D. Compare the advantages and disadvantages of the anaesthetic induction techniques for this child (8 marks)

	Gas induction (4 marks)	Rapid sequence IV induction (4 marks)
Advantages	1.	1. .... 2. ....
Disadvantages	1. .... 2. .... 3.	1. .... 2. ....

Total 20 marks

Question 12

A 74-year-old female requires laparoscopic cholecystectomy. She has no past medical history. Preoperative assessment reveals she is a current long-term smoker. You suspect she should be diagnosed with COPD.

A. Name 3 of the clinical features of COPD? (3 marks)

1. ....

2. ....

3. ....

B. You request pulmonary function tests (PFTs) to assess severity. What features on PFTs are characteristic of COPD? (2 marks)

1. ....

2. ....

C. The PFTs indicate severe COPD. What other investigations should be considered in a patient with severe COPD and why? (4 marks)

Investigation	Reason for Investigation

Note: Need to have correct test and reasoning to get each full mark.

D. You decide to refer the patient for a respiratory opinion before surgery. List 6 possible treatment modalities that are considered for optimization of this patient? (6 marks)

1. ....

2. ....

3. ....

4. ....

5. ....

6. ....

E. The patient is optimized and listed for theatre. The airway pressure is high during laparoscopy and the patient is difficult to ventilate.

Describe the mechanism of intrinsic positive end expiratory pressure (PEEPi) (1 mark)

....

....

F. Briefly describe 2 ways in which PEEPi can be recognized on a ventilator (2 marks)

1. ....

2. ....

G. What strategies can be used to reduce airway pressures in this patient, assuming a patent airway and normal equipment function? (3 marks)

1. ....

2. ....

3. ....

Exam 3 **Answers**

Many of the following questions contain more answers than there are marks allocated. This redundancy is intentional and is to ensure that a spread of possible answers by the candidate are recognized. 1 mark is awarded per correct point up to the maximum specified in each subsection.

Question 1

A 56-year-old man attends for trans-sphenoid resection of hypophyseal tumour. He has a long history of headaches and blurred vision. The diagnosis is of benign pituitary adenoma and he has clinical features of acromegaly.

A. What pathophysiology causes acromegaly? (1 mark)

1. Excess secretion of growth hormone after puberty   (1)

Note: if the disorder occurs before the growth plates have fused, as in childhood, it is called gigantism.

B. Which other hormones are secreted from the pituitary gland? (2 marks)

Location in pituitary	Hormones secreted
Anterior lobe (1 mark)	Adrenocorticotrophic hormone (ACTH) Prolactin (PRL) Follicle-stimulating hormone (FSH) Luteinizing hormone (LH) Thyroid-stimulating hormone (TSH) Melanocyte stimulating hormone (MSH) Endorphins Encephalins Note: need at least 4 anterior pituitary hormones for 1 mark. No marks for growth hormone again.
Posterior lobe (1 mark)	Antidiuretic hormone (ADH) Oxytocin Note: need both posterior pituitary hormones for one mark.

(2)

C. What are the patient specific features of acromegaly which are relevant to anaesthesia? (4 marks)

1. Increased incidence of difficult airway
2. Sleep apnoea syndrome in 50% patients
3. Large mandible and tongue
4. Overgrowth of soft tissues in the larynx and pharynx decreases the laryngeal aperture
5. May have associated recurrent laryngeal nerve palsy
6. May have goitre   (4)

D. What are the special considerations within the anaesthetic management of this patient for trans-sphenoidal hypophysectomy that you would consider in your preoperative assessment? (5 marks)

1. Consider preop indicators of difficult airway
2. Optimize coexisting hypertension
3. Clinically assess intracranial pressure (ICP) and visual function
4. Assess cardiac status (e.g. indicators of LVH/LVF/IHD) via history and ECG
5. Assess renal function, review serial U + E's
6. Check hormone assays and correct. ACTH, cortisol, TSH, and T4
7. Avoid sedative premedication
8. Consider antisialagogue
9. Check for normoglycaemia or treat diabetes   (5)

E. The surgeon asks you to facilitate a bloodless field. What can you do to help? (2 marks)

1. Ensure good venous drainage: head up tilt, endotracheal tube taped rather than tied
2. Avoid hypercapnia
3. Anaesthetic technique which obtunds/avoids hypertensive surges   (2)

F. You plan to awaken and extubate the patient immediately at the end of the procedure. What homeostatic variables must be achieved to facilitate this? (3 marks)

1. Temperature normal
2. Oxygenation adequate, respiration regular with sufficient minute ventilation
3. Normoglycaemia
4. Corticosteroid replacement   (3)

G. You plan to place the patient in HDU postoperatively. What specific management should be instituted for this patient as an adjunct to standard HDU care? (3 marks)

1. Eye movements/visual fields/acuity monitored frequently
2. Conscious level monitored frequently
3. Investigate/monitor for diabetes insipidus
4. Hormone replacement/steroid replacement/close liaison with endocrine team
5. Avoid continuous positive airway pressure (CPAP)—risk of tension pneumocephalus   (3)

Total 20 marks

Further reading

R Menon, PG Murphy, AM Lindley; Anaesthesia and pituitary disease, *Continuing Education in Anaesthesia Critical Care & Pain*, Volume 11, Issue 4, August 2011, Pages 133–137.

N Smith, P Hirsch; Pituitary disease and anaesthesia, *BJA: British Journal of Anaesthesia*, Volume 85, Issue 1, 1 July 2000, Pages 3–14.

Question 2

A 39-year-old female is listed for DIEP breast reconstruction. Her only medical history is breast cancer.

A. Outline the 2 main categories of autologous flap blood supply used in plastic surgery
(2 marks)

  1. Pedicle flap: tissue remains connected to the original donor site via an intact vascular pedicle (e.g. latissimus dorsi flap in breast reconstruction)
  2. Free flap: completely detached from the body with division of the vascular pedicle, then re-established using microvascular surgery (e.g. DIEP free flap in breast reconstruction)　(2)

B. What are the physical determinants of blood flow through a flap? (4 marks)

State their relationship to one another (1 mark)

Determinants are:

  1. Viscosity of blood
  2. Blood pressure gradient
  3. Radius of vessels
  4. Length of vessels

Relationship:

1. $Q = Pr^4\pi/8\eta L$

(Q = flow, η = viscosity, P = pressure gradient, r = radius, L = length)　(5)

Note: survival of the free flap depends on an adequate blood flow. Although blood is not a Newtonian fluid and the vessels are not rigid, the relationship is often described by the Hagen–Poiseuille equation which describes laminar flow and includes parameters which are amenable to manipulation.

C. What non-standard monitoring is considered appropriate for this procedure? (3 marks)

  1. Invasive arterial blood pressure
  2. Urine output
  3. Peripheral/skin temperature probe
  4. Cardiac output monitoring
  5. Depth of anaesthesia monitoring　(3)

D. **What are the intraoperative physiological goals targeted to improve the chances of flap survival?** (6 marks)

1. Normothermia/avoid hypothermia
2. Minimal core and peripheral/skin temperature differential
3. Normovolaemia/avoid hypovolaemia
4. Low systemic vascular resistance/peripheral vasodilatation
5. High cardiac output
6. Large pulse pressure
7. Aim normal systolic arterial pressure (systolic >100mmHg)
8. Ventilation to achieve normal pO2 and pCO2
9. Urine output 1–2ml/kg
10. Ensure optimum haematocrit 30–35% (a balance between viscosity, blood flow, and adequate oxygen carrying capacity) (6)

E. **In recovery there are concerns regarding perfusion of the flap.**

How can flap perfusion be assessed clinically at the bedside in the postoperative period? (4 marks)

1. Flap colour
2. Capillary refill time
3. Skin turgor
4. Skin temperature
5. Bleeding on pinprick
6. Transcutaneous doppler signal over perforator blood vessel) (4)

Total 20 marks

Further reading

Anaesthesia for reconstructive free flap surgery https://www.frca.co.uk/article.aspx?articleid=100376
N Nimalan, OA Branford, G Stocks; Anaesthesia for free flap breast reconstruction, *BJA Education*, Volume 16, Issue 5, 2016, Pages 162–166.

Question 3

A 67-year-old man is scheduled for laryngoscopy and biopsy for suspected carcinoma. The surgeon has requested a tubeless field so you have therefore decided to use TIVA

A. **List 5 other specific indications for TIVA** (5 marks)

1. Malignant hyperthermia
2. Long QT syndrome
3. Severe postoperative nausea and vomiting
4. Patients with anticipated difficult intubation/extubation
5. Neurosurgery

6. Neuromuscular disorders where use of volatile can be disadvantageous

7. Anaesthesia in a non-theatre environment

8. Transfer of an anaesthetised patient   (5)

B. **You are using a TCI of propofol.**

Outline the key components of a TCI device (4 marks)

1. A pump

2. A user interface to enter patient details (e.g. age, weight, height, etc.)

3. Software with a pharmacokinetic model validated for the specific drug to control infusion rate

4. Communication between control unit and pump hardware

5. Visual and audible safety alarms   (4)

C. **List 2 pharmacokinetic adult models used for propofol** (2 marks)

1. Marsh

2. Modified Marsh

3. Schnider

4. Eleveld   (2)

D. **Describe the three-compartment pharmacokinetic model for a bolus of propofol** (5 marks)

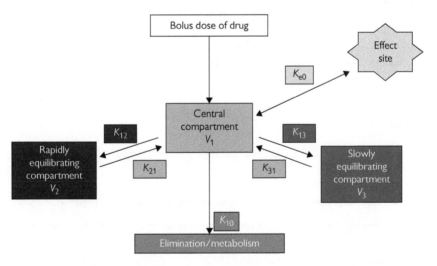

This figure was published in *BJA Education*, 16(3), Z Al-Rifai and D Mulvey. Principles of total intravenous anaesthesia: basic pharmacokinetics and model descriptions. 92-97. Copyright © 2016, with permission from Elsevier Ltd., British Journal of Anaesthesia and The Royal College of Anaesthetists.

1. After an intravenous bolus of a drug the plasmas concentration shows an exponential decline in 3 distinct phases

2. This is explained by the distribution of the drug in the central compartment V1 (plasma) and 2 other peripheral compartments

3. V2 represents well perfused tissue such as muscle so distribution is relatively fast

4. V3 represents poorly perfused tissue such as fat so distribution and redistribution from this compartment is slow

5. It is the plasma concentration that influences the effect site concentration

Note: 5 marks given for the figure completed or written points (5)

E. Describe how a TCI device ensures a steady state concentration of a drug (4 marks)

1. A bolus/elimination/transfer (BET) principle is used to achieve a steady state plasma concentration

2. Initially a bolus is given to fill the central compartment V1

3. The subsequent infusion rate compensates for the distribution to compartments V2 and V3 and elimination from V1

4. When all 3 compartments reach steady state concentration the infusion rate decreases to match elimination from V1 only

5. Depending on pharmacokinetic model used, patient details such as sex and weight are entered to inform targeted plasma concentration

6. The system calculates the bolus and infusion rate required to achieve this. Calculations are repeated regularly, and infusion rate adjusted to achieve targeted plasma concentration (4)

Total 20 marks

Further reading

Z Al-Rifai, D Mulvey; Principles of total intravenous anaesthesia: basic pharmacokinetics and model descriptions, *BJA Education*, Volume 16, Issue 3, March 2016, Pages 92–97.

Association of Anaesthetists; *Safe Practice of Total Intravenous Anaesthesia* 2018 https://anaesthetists.org/ Home/Resources-publications/Guidelines/Safe-practice-of-total-intravenous-anaesthesia-TIVA-2018

Question 4

You and your consultant are about to perform brainstem death testing on a 64-year-old woman in the ICU.

A. List 4 'red flags' when diagnostic caution is advised for brainstem death testing? (4 marks)

1. Testing less than 24 hours after presentation where aetiology is primarily anoxic damage

2. Testing less than 6 hours after loss of last brainstem reflex

3. Hypothermia—temperature must be >36°C

4. Patient known to have a neuromuscular disorder

5. Steroids have been administered for a space occupying lesion

6. Prolonged fentanyl infusion used

7. Aetiology primarily located to brainstem or posterior fossa (4)

B. **Describe how you would perform the apnoea test as part of the brainstem death testing?**
(6 marks)

1. Preoxygenate the patient with FiO_2 1.0
2. Allow $PaCO_2$ to rise by reducing minute ventilation
3. Confirm $PaCO_2$ >6kPa and pH <7.4 on an arterial blood gas
4. Either use a CPAP circuit (Mapleson C) or disconnect from ventilator and administer oxygen via catheter in the trachea at a rate of 6L/min. It is not recommended to perform tests while on mechanical ventilation
5. Observe for no spontaneous ventilation for a minimum of 5 minutes following disconnection
6. Confirm $PaCO_2$ has increased >0.5kPa from starting $PaCO_2$
7. Maintain oxygenation and cardiovascular stability throughout testing
8. Perform manual recruitment before resuming mechanical ventilation   (6)

C. **You have completed both sets of brainstem death tests, confirmed death by neurological criteria and spoken with the family. The patient is going to proceed to organ donation. She currently has an arterial blood pressure of 84/39mmHg and a CVP of 3 mmHg.**

Outline your cardiovascular targets for this patient to maximize donor potential (3 marks)

Heart rate range (bpm) (1 mark)	60–120
Mean arterial pressure range (mmHg) (1 mark)	>75 and <95
CVP range (mmHg) (1 mark)	6–10

(3)

D. **How would you achieve these cardiovascular targets?** (2 marks)

1. Careful fluid resuscitation—colloid or crystalloid to euvolaemia
2. Vasopressin is first-line agent to restore vascular tone
3. Noradrenaline infusion can be used but should be weaned off and vasopressin used in preference as can affect suitability of heart for transplantation due to myocardial damage   (2)

E. **This patient has a urine output of over 400ml/hour.**

What biochemical features would confirm the diagnosis of Diabetes Insipidus? (2 marks)

1. High serum sodium/hypernatraemia >145mmol/L
2. Increased serum osmolality >295mOsm/kg H20
3. Decreased urine osmolality <450mOsm/kg H20   (2)

F. Outline your management of the main endocrine abnormalities that occur after brainstem death (3 marks)

1. Methylprednisolone 15mg/kg every 24 hours
2. Insulin infusion to maintain normoglycaemia
3. Desmopressin and/or vasopressin to treat diabetes insipidus
4. Thyroid hormone (T3) replacement (3)

Total 20 marks

Further reading

JK Gordon, J McKinlay; Physiological changes after brain stem death and management of the heart-beating donor, *Continuing Education in Anaesthesia Critical Care & Pain*, Volume 12, Issue 5, October 2012, Pages 225–229.

The Faculty of Intensive Care Medicine; Form for the diagnosis of death using neurological criteria, FICM https://www.ficm.ac.uk/sites/default/files/form_for_the_diagnosis_of_death_using_neurological_criteria_-_long_version_nov_2019_003.pdf

Question 5

A 32-year-old woman attends for pelvic laparoscopy. She weighs 70kg and her BMI is 35. Her medical history is severe reflux. She had generalized muscular ache following administration of suxamethonium during a previous anaesthetic. Her medication is omeprazole 20mg bd and the oral contraceptive pill. You decide to use rocuronium to facilitate intubation.

A. Give 5 other advantages of using rocuronium instead of suxamethonium for a rapid sequence induction (5 marks)

1. Longer time available for intubation
2. Can be used safely in burns and neurological injures
3. Can be reversed in can't intubate, can't ventilate scenario
4. Can be stored at room temperature (although reduced shelf life—see note)
5. Reduced histamine release
6. No risk of malignant hyperthermia (MH)
7. No clinical significance in the subpopulation with cholinesterase deficiency (5)

Note: rocuronium can be stored in a cupboard in temperatures up to 30°C for 12 weeks. After this time it should be discarded. Do not refrigerate after removal from fridge.

B. What dose of rocuronium would you use for a rapid sequence induction in this patient? (1 mark)

1–1.2mg/kg × 70kg = 70–84mg rocuronium (1)

C. Describe the pharmacodynamic principle which accounts for rocuronium's more rapid onset of action when compared to vecuronium? (2 marks)

1. Rocuronium is a lower potency drug (weaker antagonist at the neuromuscular junction) and is given in a larger dose for the same maximal effect (e.g. 5 times the dose of vecuronium is required for the same effect)
2. The presence of many more molecules in the larger dose thus results in a larger diffusion gradient and faster saturation of the postsynaptic receptors—hence a more rapid onset   (2)

Note: no association has been established with regard to its lipid solubility or protein binding as regards speed of onset.

D. Give 2 processes by which the effects of rocuronium can be terminated at the end of the procedure (2 marks)

1. Removal of drug from circulation
2. Increase in concentration of acetylcholine (competitive agonism)   (2)

E. Explain the pharmacology of each method (4 marks)

Process 1 (removal of drug from circulation)

1. Occurs with sugammadex by irreversible encapsulation of lipophilic rocuronium molecules; a process known as chelation
2. As the free concentration of rocuronium in plasma reduces, further dissociation of the drug from the ACh receptors results by diffusion down a concentration gradient   (2)

Process 2 (increase in concentration of acetylcholine)

1. Neostigmine hydrolyses acetylcholinesterase enzymes which allow the concentration of acetylcholine in the neuromuscular junction to build up, exceed the concentration of ACh and occupy more receptors
2. This allows development of a postsynaptic excitatory potential which will eventually reach the threshold required to trigger an action potential   (2)

F. What dose of sugammadex would you precalculate for immediate reversal of rocuronium in the event of a failed intubation in this patient? (1 mark)

70kg × 16mg/kg = 1120mg   (1)

G. 30 minutes later in the recovery room the patient is hypotensive and is to return to theatre with suspected intra-abdominal bleeding.

Give 3 drug options available to facilitate laryngoscopy conditions during repeat intubation (3 marks)

1. Suxamethonium
2. Opioid coadministration (e.g. alfentanil or remifentanil)
3. Atracurium or cis-atracurium
4. Use rocuronium again. Although repeat use within 24 hours is not recommended, earlier use still causes neuromuscular blockade although the speed of onset, the dose required, and

resulting efficacy is variable. Rapid onset is unlikely, even in a traditional rapid sequence dose (3)

H. What postoperative advice would you give to this patient regarding their administration of sugammadex? (2 marks)

1. Sugammadex may decrease the effectiveness of hormonal contraceptive for up to 7 days
2. The patient should use alternate methods of contraception during this period
3. Continue to take your oral contraceptive pill (OCP) daily during this period
4. Dispensation of written information regarding implications for contraception

(2)

Total 20 marks

Further reading

D Chambers, M Paulden, F Paton, et al.; Sugammadex for reversal of neuromuscular block after rapid sequence intubation: a systematic review and economic assessment, *BJA: British Journal of Anaesthesia*, Volume 105, Issue 5, November 2010, Pages 568–575.

G Cammu, P-J de Kam, K De Graeve, M van den Heuvel; Repeat dosing of rocuronium 1.2 mg kg−1 after reversal of neuromuscular block by sugammadex 4.0 mg kg−1 in anaesthetized healthy volunteers: a modelling-based pilot study, *BJA: British Journal of Anaesthesia*, Volume 105, Issue 4, October 2010, Pages 487–492.

R Khirwadkar, JM Hunter; Neuromuscular physiology and pharmacology: an update, *Continuing Education in Anaesthesia Critical Care & Pain*, Volume 12, Issue 5, October 2012, Pages 237–244.

TE Peck, SA Hill; *Pharmacology for Anaesthesia and Intensive Care* 4th edition. Cambridge: Cambridge University Press, 2014.

J Roy, F Varin; Physicochemical properties of neuromuscular blocking agents and their impact on the pharmacy-kinetic and pharmacodynamic relationship, *BJA; British Journal Anaesthesia*, Volume 93, Issue 2, August 2004, Pages 241–248.

Question 6

A company representative attends your department one lunchtime to showcase their new ultrasound machine.

A. Give 4 examples each, of diagnostic and therapeutic uses of ultrasound in anaesthetic and critical care practice? (8 marks)

Diagnostic

1. Ascites detection
2. Pleural fluid/pneumothorax detection
3. FAST scanning (focused assessment surgical trauma)
4. Cardiac output, tamponade detection
5. Middle cerebral artery flow in neonates (4)

Therapeutic

1. Safe guidance for central venous catheter insertion (feeding, dialysis) and arterial line insertion
2. Safe practice of peripheral nerve blocks
3. Lumbar spine assessment prior to central neuraxial block: intervertebral spaces, midline, and depths
4. High frequency ultrasound treatment of acute pain
5. Identification of peripheral veins in morbidly obese
6. Identification of sacral hiatus prior to caudal block
7. Identification of the cricothyroid membrane prior to cannulation (4)

B. **What is the Doppler effect?** (2 marks)

The Doppler effect is the change in frequency (1 mark) of a wave (or other periodic event) for an observer moving relative to its source (1 mark) (2)

C. **Give 2 applications of the Doppler effect used in echocardiography** (2 marks)

1. To determine direction and speed of blood flow (across valves or through ASD/VSD)
2. To determine cardiac output (2)

D. **What information can echocardiography provide in a haemodynamically unstable patient?** (8 marks)

1. Myocardial function: to assess ventricular contractility and detect regional wall motion abnormalities
2. Ejection fraction
3. Can measure end diastolic filling volume/assess hypovolaemic state
4. Valvular dysfunction (regurgitation/prolapse/vegetations)
5. Confirm the diagnosis of cardiac tamponade or pericardial effusion
6. Diagnosis of cardiomegaly
7. Can determine the size of cardiac chambers
8. Can measure and observe the heart rate and arrythmia
9. Thrombo-embolic disease: indirect diagnosis of pulmonary embolism (RV strain), visualize any intracardiac thrombosis or atrial myxoma
10. Rapid assessment of thoracic trauma
11. Diagnosis of aortic dissection (8)

Note: In some instances, there are better options for the diagnosis of the aforementioned states but echocardiography does not usually require transfer and can be performed at the bedside

Total 20 marks

Further reading

A Roscoe, T Strang; Echocardiography in intensive care, *Continuing Education in Anaesthesia Critical Care & Pain*, Volume 8, Issue 2, April 2008, Pages 46–49.

Question 7

A 59-year-old woman has presented with gradual onset leg weakness and now has difficulty walking. She is normally fit and well but had a self-limiting episode of gastroenteritis 3 weeks ago. She takes no regular medication.

A. List the classic clinical features of GBS (5 marks)

1. Progressive ascending motor weakness
2. Hypo or areflexia
3. Sensory symptoms
4. Pain, often in the pelvic girdle area
5. If ascends to respiratory muscles respiratory failure results
6. Facial nerve palsies
7. Bulbar palsy—difficulty swallowing
8. Ophthalmoplegia
9. Autonomic dysfunction—labile blood pressure, arrhythmia, urinary retention (5)

B. What specific investigations, with their findings, would support a diagnosis of GBS? (6 marks)

1. Lumbar puncture—raised protein level, normal cell count, and glucose
2. Infection screen—positive serology for campylobacter, CMV, ABV, herpes simplex, mycoplasma pneumonia, HIV
3. Stool culture—positive for campylobacter
4. Antiganglioside antibodies—positive levels of AntiGM1 found in 25%
5. ESR—raised level
6. Nerve conduction studies—demyelinating pattern
7. Computed tomography (CT) brain—negative for other causes of symptoms

Note: Must have 3 investigations with findings for marks (6)

C. The patient is admitted to HDU and she is investigated for suspected GBS. However, over the last 48 hours she develops symmetrical arm weakness as well. Today she is struggling to cough and swallow and her respiratory rate has increased to 32 breaths/min. Her PaO_2 is 8.9kPA on 70% oxygen.

You decide she needs ventilatory support.

What specific modifications would you make to your induction and intubating technique for this patient? (2 marks)

1. She will need a rapid sequence induction as she has symptoms of bulbar palsy
2. Suxamethonium is contraindicated as it may precipitate hyperkalaemia, therefore 1–1.2mg/kg rocuronium is a suggested alternative
3. Use an induction sparing coagent such as alfentanil and exercise caution with induction agent to minimize cardiovascular instability
4. Also care with vasopressors as response may be exaggerated with autonomic instability (2)

D. You intubate without incident. She is now ventilated and fully monitored, with an arterial and central line, in ICU. Outline your ongoing specific (2 marks) and supportive management (5 marks) for this patient.

Specific

1. Immunoglobulin therapy considered on specialist advice
2. Plasma exchange considered on specialist advice

Note: No marks given for steroids (2)

Supportive

1. Often ventilation prolonged, consider early tracheostomy
2. DVT prophylaxis as high risk of thromboembolic disease
3. Treat autonomic instability, care with suctioning of trachea
4. Enteral feeding and nutritional support. Higher incidence of paralytic ileus so may need prokinetic therapy added
5. Neuropathic pain very common—careful assessment and treatment
6. High incidence of depression—monitor and treat
7. Physiotherapy—chest and rehabilitation of global weakness
8. Careful limb positioning (5)

Total 20 marks

Further reading

S Marsh, A Pittard; Neuromuscular disorders and anaesthesia. Part 2: specific neuromuscular disorders, *Continuing Education in Anaesthesia Critical Care & Pain*, Volume 11, Issue 4, August 2011, Pages 119–123.
KJC Richards, AT Cohen; Guillain-Barré syndrome, *BJA CEPD Reviews*, Volume 3, Issue 2, April 2003, Pages 46–49.

Question 8

You receive a trauma call to the ED. A 22-year-old man was the driver of a car involved in a high-speed road traffic collision. He has multiple injuries.

A. You suspect an immediate life-threatening thoracic injury. List 5 treatable causes of this found on primary survey (5 marks)

1. Airway obstruction or airway rupture
2. Tension pneumothorax (must specify tension)
3. Open pneumothorax (must specify open)
4. Massive haemothorax (must specify massive)
5. Flail chest
6. Cardiac tamponade (5)

B. **What immediate diagnostic imaging is appropriate for diagnosing chest trauma?** (2 marks)

1. Chest X-ray
2. Extended focused assessment with sonography for trauma (eFAST)
3. Immediate CT (only in absence of severe respiratory compromise, if responding to resuscitation, or in those whose haemodynamic status is normal) (2)

C. **Primary survey is now complete. The patient is breathing spontaneously but not moving his arms or legs. A C5 cervical spine injury is suspected.**

What are the clinical features on examination of an acute C5 cervical spine injury? (5 marks)

1. Neck pain
2. Loss of pain/sensation below the level of injury
3. Diaphragmatic breathing
4. Hypotension and bradycardia
5. Warm and dilated peripherally
6. Priapism
7. Flaccidity
8. Areflexia (5)

D. **Describe the specific modifications to airway management during a rapid sequence induction of anaesthesia for this patient** (4 marks)

1. Removal of hard collar and blocks preinduction of anaesthesia
2. Manual in-line stabilization (MILS)
3. 2-handed cricoid pressure from assistant (with 2nd hand supporting c-spine posteriorly)
4. Attention to minimal C-spine movement during laryngoscopy
5. Difficult airway equipment available (4)

Notes: No individual airway technique is superior, it is more important to avoid hypoxia and use familiar methods. Despite direct and indirect intubation techniques and cricoid pressure all being associated with spinal movement, this movement is unlikely to result in neurological injury providing reasonable care is taken.

E. One month later the patient is transferred to a spinal injuries unit.

Briefly describe these clinical syndromes resulting from spinal cord injury (4 marks)

Syndrome	Description
Anterior spinal artery syndrome (2 marks)	1. Single artery supplies the anterior 2/3 of the cord—transection therefore produces sparing of the dorsal columns 2. Paralysis and loss of pain and temperature sensation 3. Preservation of proprioception, fine touch, and vibration
Brown-Séquard syndrome (2 marks)	1. Lateral cord damage 2. Ipsilateral loss of motor function and fine touch/proprioception/ vibration. 3. Contralateral loss of pain and temperature sensation

(4)

Total 20 marks

Further reading

A Blyth; Thoracic trauma, ABC of Major Trauma, 4th Edition, *British Medical Journal*, Volume 348, 2014, bmj. g1137.

S Bonner, C Smith; Initial management of acute spinal cord injury, *Continuing Education in Anaesthesia Critical Care & Pain*, Volume 13, Issue 6, December 2013, Pages 224–31.

NICE Guideline. Major trauma: assessment and initial management. 2016 https://www.nice.org.uk/guidance/ng39

Question 9

You are to anaesthetise a 78-year-old woman for an elective right total hip replacement. She weighs 51kg and has a past medical history including stable angina, hypertension, COPD, and peripheral vascular disease. You plan a spinal anaesthetic with a target-controlled infusion of propofol (TCI) for deep sedation.

A. Define IPH? (1 mark)

IPH is defined as a core body temperature <36.0°c (1)

B. This patient's temperature on arrival in the theatre suite is 35.4°C.

List 5 risk factors for the development of IPH in this patient? (5 marks)

1. High American Society of Anesthesiologists (ASA) grade/multiple comorbidities
2. Combined regional and general anaesthesia/sedation planned
3. Major surgery
4. Low BMI
5. Elderly

6. Low preoperative temperature <36°C
7. Duration of surgery: long procedures greater risk than short procedures, but procedures lasting an hour are most at risk
8. Cold theatre environment/laminar flow theatre
9. Large wound for heat loss and bleeding   (5)

C. Describe in detail 4 major consequences and the associated pathophysiology of IPH that may impact the morbidity and mortality of patients (8 marks)

Major consequence of IPH (4 marks)	Pathophysiology (4 marks)
1. Increased surgical site infection	1. Due to decreases blood flow and oxygen flux to the tissues
2. Altered drug metabolism	2. Hepatic metabolism reduced leading to prolonged action of opiates, propofol, and neuromuscular blockers. Also decreased maximum aerobic capacity (MAC) and slower recovery form inhalational anaesthesia
3. Increased bleeding risk and higher transfusion requirements	3. Impaired platelet function and impaired coagulation cascade
4. Increased risk of cardiac events	4. Increased postoperative catecholamine release leading to increased arterial blood pressure and myocardial workload
5. Shivering	5. Increases skeletal muscle oxygen demand causes an increase in cardiac workload. This can compound cardiac ischaemia. Also increases postoperative pain

Note: Any 4 of the 5 consequences with correct pathophysiology for full 8 marks.   (8)

D. **Outline your management of this patient's temperature before and during surgery** (6 marks)

1. Active warming should be started preoperatively as she is high risk for IPH
2. Patient should not be transferred, or anaesthesia induced until temperature >36°C
3. Ensure ambient theatre temperature >21°C
4. Active forced air warming
5. Warm intravenous fluids
6. Humidify respiratory gases
7. Measure temperature every 30 mins and titrate active warming as required
8. Insert continual core temperature probe   (6)

Total 20 marks

Further reading

NICE Guideline (CG65) Hypothermia: Prevention and management in adults undergoing surgery. Published April 2008. Updated December 2016 https://www.nice.org.uk/guidance/cg65

Question 10

A 32-year-old woman, Para 2 + 0 is having a caesarean section under spinal anaesthesia.

The baby and placenta have been delivered successfully but there is ongoing bleeding of approximately 800mls so far.

A. **List 4 main causes of primary PPH** (4 marks)

1. Uterine atony
2. Retained products
3. Genital tract trauma
4. Coagulopathy—inherited or acquired   (4)

Note: this is the '4T's' of PPH—tone, tissue, trauma, and thrombin

B. Complete the table of drugs used to treat uterine atony as directed. Give their doses and routes of administration. List their mechanisms of action and common side effects (12 marks)

Drug	Dose and route of administration	Mechanism of action	Side effects
Oxytocin (3 marks)	Slow intravenous bolus of 5IU repeated if required. Or commence IV infusion, typically using 10 IU/h for 4 hours	Direct agonist on myometrial oxytocin receptors causing contraction	Vasodilatation Hypotension Tachycardia
Ergometrine (3 marks)	Typical dose of 500mcg can be given either intravenously (slowly) or intramuscularly	Acts on alpha adrenergic receptors in uterus to cause contraction	Nausea and vomiting Increased blood pressure Bronchospasm
Carboprost (3 marks)	0.25mg dose can be given intramuscularly, repeated to a total dose of 2mg. Intramyometrial administration has a more rapid onset but is an 'off-label' use	Synthetic Prostaglandin F2 Alpha analogue causing uterine contraction	Nausea Bronchospasm
Misoprostol (3 marks)	Can be used rectally, orally, or sublingually The recommended dose is 800mcg	A prostaglandin E1 analogue causing uterine contraction	Nausea Bronchospasm

(12)

C. Despite the appropriate administration of uterotonics over the last 20 minutes and administration of 2L of crystalloid, the bleeding is ongoing with blood loss now at 1.5L.

Outline the next steps in your management of this patient (4 marks)

1. Activate major haemorrhage protocol
2. Alert senior staff
3. Give 15L oxygen via trauma mask
4. Administer tranexamic acid 1g
5. Establish further wide bore access/2nd large cannula and take bloods for FBC, COAG, U&Es
6. Request blood products—crossmatch 4–6 units and fresh frozen plasma

7. Prepare for conversion to GA (RSI)
8. Consider invasive monitoring
9. Ensure normothermia with active warming
10. Consider repeat antibiotic

Note: Must have activate major haemorrhage protocol as one of the answers for award of full marks

(4)

Total 20 marks

Further reading

E Mavrides, S Allard, E Chandraharan, et al. on behalf of the Royal College of Obstetricians and Gynaecologists. Prevention and management of postpartum haemorrhage. *BJOG: An International Journal of Obstetrics and Gynaecology*, Volume 124, 2016, Pages e106–e149.

Question 11

A 6-year-old girl requires elective tonsillectomy. She has no significant medical history.

A. Briefly describe 2 indications for paediatric tonsillectomy? (2 marks)

1. Recurrent proven sore throats due to bacterial tonsillitis
2. Persisting, disabling symptoms preventing normal function (e.g. going to school)
3. Obstructive sleep apnoea symptoms

(2)

B. Regarding the choice of airway technique for this case, what are the advantages of each below?

	Laryngeal mask airway (LMA) (3 marks)	Tracheal Intubation (3 marks)
Advantages	1. No laryngoscopy required which is less stimulating 2. Smooth emergence, minimal coughing 3. No paralysis required 4. LMA left *in situ* until awake provides some degree of protection of the larynx from soiling by blood	1. Secure airway 2. Good surgical access 3. Laryngoscopy grade known 4. Finer control of ventilation/CO_2

(6)

C. She re-presents as an emergency 12 hours postoperatively with bleeding from the tonsillar bed. The ENT surgeon wishes to expedite her return to theatre.

List 4 clinical challenges pertaining to this case (4 marks)

1. Hypovolaemia
2. Difficulty in estimation of volume lost due to blood swallowed
3. Full stomach (with blood)
4. Difficult airway/laryngoscopy view obscured by bleeding
5. Anxious child and parents
6. Recent general anaesthesia
7. Securing IV access   (4)

D. Compare the advantages and disadvantages of the anaesthetic induction techniques for this child (8 marks)

	Gas induction (4 marks)	**Rapid sequence IV induction** (4 marks)
Advantages	1. Respiration is maintained as not paralysed	1. Less distressing, quick procedure 2. Reduced risk of aspiration, airway secured quickly 3. Familiar to most anaesthetists
Disadvantages	1. Prolonged time to achieve adequate depth 2. Risk of aspiration from unprotected airway 3. More distressing to the child 4. Unfamiliar	1. Difficult to judge precalculated doses in hypovolaemic child 2. Reduced time available for successful intubation 3. IV/IO access required from outset

(8)

Total 20 marks

Further reading

R Ravi, T Howell; Anaesthesia for paediatric ear, nose, and throat surgery, *Continuing Education in Anaesthesia Critical Care & Pain*, Volume 7, Issue 2, 1 April 2007, Pages 33–37.

SIGN Guideline 117: Management of sore throat and indications for tonsillectomy 2010. https://www.guidelines.co.uk/infection/sign-sore-throat-guideline/455177.article

Question 12

A 74-year-old female requires laparoscopic cholecystectomy. She has no past medical history. Preoperative assessment reveals she is a current long-term smoker. You suspect she should be diagnosed with COPD.

A. Name 3 of the clinical features of COPD? (3 marks)

1. Exertional breathlessness
2. Chronic cough
3. Regular sputum production
4. Frequent bronchitis or wheeze during winter months (3)

B. You request PFTs to assess severity. What features on PFTs are characteristic of COPD? (2 marks)

1. Reduced FEV1 and FVC
2. FEV:FVC <0.7 (2)

C. The PFTs indicate severe COPD. What other investigations should be considered in a patient with severe COPD and why? (4 marks)

Investigation	Reason for investigation
1. ECG or echo	Evidence of right-sided heart disease (cor pulmonale)
2. Full blood count	Detection of polycythaemia or raised white cell count for intercurrent infection
3. Chest X-ray	Extensive bullous disease might indicate risk of pneumothorax
4. Arterial blood gas	$PaCO_2$ >5.9kPa and PaO_2 <7.9kPa predicts worse outcome

Note: Both investigation and reason are required for one mark. Other investigations might be considered but are less common than those stated. (4)

D. You decide to refer the patient for a respiratory opinion before surgery. List 6 possible treatment modalities that are considered for optimization of this patient? (6 marks)

1. Smoking cessation
2. Pulmonary rehabilitation programme
3. Inhaled bronchodilators: short/long acting beta$_2$ agonist, long acting muscarinic antagonist
4. Inhaled corticosteroids
5. Oral steroids (usually intermittent)
6. Oral theophylline
7. Long-term oxygen therapy

8. Preoperative chest physiotherapy

9. Surgery—bullae reduction (6)

E. The patient is optimized and listed for theatre. The airway pressure is high during laparoscopy and the patient is difficult to ventilate.

Describe the mechanism of intrinsic positive end expiratory pressure (PEEPi) (1 mark)

Lower airway obstruction results in the next inhalation occurring before expiration of the previous breath is complete, and leads to 'breath stacking' or 'air trapping' and the development of intrinsic positive end expiratory pressure, Intrinsic PEEP (PEEPi)

F. Briefly describe 2 ways in which PEEPi can be recognized on a ventilator? (2 marks)

1. Capnography trace that does not reach a plateau

2. Expiratory flow on the flowmeter has not reached zero

3. Measurement of PEEPi (2)

G. What strategies can be used to reduce airway pressures in this patient, assuming a patent airway and normal equipment function? (3 marks)

1. Reduce respiratory rate or lengthen I:E ratio

2. Chest suction via endotracheal (ET) tube

3. Permissive hypercapnia while avoiding hypoxia

4. Ensure no iatrogenic pneumothorax and treat as necessary

5. Consider choice of volatile anaesthesia—sevoflurane probably preferable to desflurane for airway pressure management

6. Consider wheeze and if present administer a bronchodilator/deepening sevoflurane volatile anaesthesia

7. Convert to open cholecystectomy procedure (3)

Total 20 marks

Further reading

A Lumb, C Biercamp; Chronic obstructive pulmonary disease and anaesthesia, *Continuing Education in Anaesthesia Critical Care & Pain*, Volume 14, Issue 1, February 2014, Pages 1–5.

Exam 4   **Questions**

Exam 4 contains 12 selected Constructed Response Questions (CRQs) balanced across the intermediate curriculum, reflecting the Final Examination of the Diploma of Fellowship of the Royal College of Anaesthetists (FRCA) exam. We recommend attempting these questions under exam conditions. **Please limit/contain your answer to/within the dotted lines given for each question.**

Question 1

A 67-year-old patient is on the trauma list for emergency surgery for fractured neck of femur. He was fitted with a permanent pacemaker 5 years ago, after suffering blackouts. His pacemaker code is DDI.

A. Describe what each letter of this pacemaker code denotes? (3 marks)

....

....

....

B. This is the patient's electrocardiogram (ECG) on admission. What information about the pacemaker can be deduced from this? (3 marks)

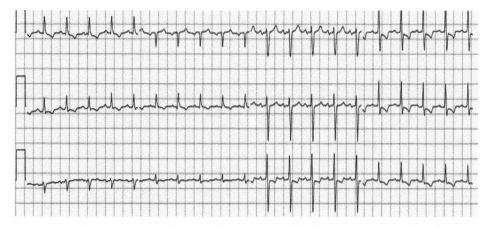

Reproduced from *Diagnosis and Treatment in Internal Medicine*, Patrick Davey and David Sprigings, Figure 111.1. Copyright Oxford University Press, 2011. Reproduced with permission of the Licensor through PLSclear.

....

....

....

C. You decide to change the pacemaker to fixed rate pacing.

What pacemaker code denotes fixed rate pacing? (1 mark)

....

D. What is the major concern if this pacemaker is subject to electrical interference? (2 marks)

....

....

E. What information do positions 4 and 5 of the pacemaker code denote? (2 marks)

....

....

F. Describe what each position (1–4) of an implantable defibrillation device code denotes (4 marks)

1. ....

2. ....

3. ....

4. ....

G. How would you advise the theatre team in the safe use of monopolar diathermy? (3 marks)

1. ....

2. ....

3. ....

H. State which anaesthetic technique you would use for this patient (1 mark) and why (1 mark)

....

....

Total 20 marks

Question 2

A 4-year-old boy is listed for strabismus surgery as a day case.

A. List the general (4 marks) and specific (4 marks) anaesthetic issues.

General considerations

1. ....

2. ....

3. ....

4. ....

Specific to this procedure

1. ....

2. ....

3. ....

4. ....

B. How would you manage profound bradycardia during surgical traction? (3 marks)

1. ....

2. ....

3. ....

C. For each of these 3 common postoperative problems, complete the table with the relevant management strategies (9 marks)

Post-op problem	Management 1 (3 marks)	Management 2 (3 marks)	Management 3 (3 marks)
PONV			
Pain			
Recovery room distress			

Total 20 marks

Question 3

A 52-year-old woman is having a right nephrectomy. She has a past medical history of hypertension for which she takes atenolol. Induction and intubation with propofol and rocuronium were straightforward. You transfer her into theatre and administer prophylactic gentamicin. Twenty minutes later, as the abdomen is being prepped her blood pressure drops to 79/32, her heart rate is 132bpm, and her airway pressures increase. You suspect anaphylaxis.

A. Outline your immediate management (4 marks)

B. Outline your secondary management (3 marks)

C. The patient's blood pressure remains at 75/42mmHg. You administer a further fluid bolus. What other secondary agents would you consider to treat the refractory hypotension? (2 marks)

D. In the NAP6 study what are the 3 most common causative agents of perioperative anaphylaxis? (3 marks)

....

....

....

E. Complete the following table with the different hypersensitivity reactions (8 marks)

Type	Description of immune response (4 marks)	Example (4 marks)
1		
2		
3		
4		

Total 20 marks

Question 4

A 52-year-old man is ventilated in the intensive care unit (ICU). He presented 4 days ago with severe community acquired pneumonia. You now suspect he has acute respiratory distress syndrome (ARDS).

A. Detail the current criteria for the diagnosis of ARDS (8 marks)

B. Describe the pathophysiology of ARDS (4 marks)

C. Complete the table to describe each of the **3** phases of ARDS (3 marks)

Phase	Pathophysiological description
Acute/exudative (1 mark)	
Proliferative/subacute (1 mark)	
Chronic/fibrotic (1 mark)	

D. What specific strategies can be used in the management of ARDS to optimize ventilation and oxygenation? (3 marks)

1. ....

2. ....

3. ....

E. List 2 beneficial effects of the prone position in severe ARDS? (2 marks)

1. ....

2. ....

Total 20 marks

Question 5

A patient attends the chronic pain clinic with facial pain. Her GP has told her he thinks she has trigeminal neuralgia (TN).

A. Give 5 characteristics of the pain that supports a diagnosis of TN? (5 marks)

1. ....

2. ....

3. ....

4. ....

5. ....

B. Give 4 differential diagnoses (4 marks)

1. ....

2. ....

3. ....

4. ....

C. What other conditions is TN associated with? (3 marks)

1. ....

2. ....

3. ....

D. What drugs would you use to treat TN? (3 marks)

1. ....

2. ....

3. ....

E. What non-pharmacological treatments are available for TN? (3 marks)

1. ....

2. ....

3. ....

4. ....

5. ....

F. If left untreated, what is the natural prognosis of the condition? (1 mark)

1. ....

G. What is the incidence of TN in the UK? Please select your answer (1 mark)

1 in 1,000   1 in 10,000   1 in 100,000

Total 20 marks

Question 6

A 61-year-old woman with endometrial cancer is listed for total abdominal hysterectomy and bilateral salpingo-ophorectomy with pelvic lymphadenectomy. Her medical history is type 2 diabetes mellitus and asthma. Her medication is metformin, gliclazide, and salbutamol. She is a long-term smoker. Her body mass index (BMI) is 48Kg/m^2.

A. What class of obesity is this patient in? (1 mark)

1. ....

B. Briefly describe the specific preoperative concerns which must be considered in this patient? (5 marks)

1. ....

2. ....

3. ....

4. ....

5. ....

C. Define the following terms considered when administering anaesthetic drugs to obese patients (4 marks)

Total body weight (TBW) (1 mark)	
Ideal body weight (IBW) (1 mark)	
Lean body weight (LBW) (1 mark)	
Adjusted Body Weight (ABW) (1 mark)	

D. What are the principles of delivering safe general anaesthesia for this patient assuming risk of sleep disordered breathing? (5 marks)

1. ....

2. ....

3. ....

4. ....

5. ....

E. What local anaesthesia based analgesic options may be considered for this case? (4 marks)

1. ....

2. ....

3. ....

4. ....

5. ....

F. What anatomical landmark indicates an ideal ramped position before induction of general anaesthesia? (1 mark)

....

Question 7

A. Please detail the 5 levels of the evidence hierarchy (5 marks)

1. ....

2. ....

3. ....

4. ....

5. ....

B. Give 4 types of bias you must be aware of, and state how can they be avoided when carrying out research? (8 marks)

1. ....

   ....

2. ....

   ....

3. ....

   ....

4. ....

   ....

C. How can results be misleading despite a double blind RCT? (2 marks)

....

....

....

....

D. What aspects should you pay particular attention to when appraising a paper? (5 marks)

1. ....

2. ....

3. ....

4. ....

5. ....

Total 20 marks

Question 8

You anaesthetise a 19-year-old woman for bimaxillary surgery. She has no significant past medical or drug history.

A. What specifically is bimaxillary surgery? (1 mark).

....

....

B. What are the common indications for this surgery which are relevant to the anaesthetist? (2 marks)

1. ....

2. ....

C. What are the main airway considerations for this case? (3 marks)

1. ....

2. ....

3. ....

D. Following successful intubation you insert a throat pack.

Describe 5 steps that are taken to ensure the throat pack is not retained in error following completion of surgery and anaesthesia? (5 marks)

1. ....

2. ....

3. ....

4. ....

5. ....

E. What techniques can be used to minimize bleeding during this operation? (2 marks)

1. ....

2. ....

3. ....

4. ....

F. The patient has intramedullary fixation (IMF) with elastics in place at cessation of surgery.

What measures are taken to ensure airway safety during emergence from anaesthesia and in the early postoperative period for this situation? (7 marks)

	Airway safety measures
Emergence (4 marks)	1. ....
	2. ....
	3. ....
	4. ....
Postoperative (3 marks)	1. ....
	2. ....
	3. ....

Total 20 marks

Question 9

You assess a 24-year-old rugby player for repair of rotator cuff in his right shoulder. He weighs 110kg and is 185cm tall. He is right-handed.

A. Name 4 nerves that need to be blocked to provide analgesia for rotator cuff repair? (4 marks)

1. ....

2. ....

3. ....

4. ....

B. What are the benefits of the interscalene approach to the brachial plexus in this case?
(4 marks)

1. ....

2. ....

3. ....

4. ....

C. Complete the table by listing 6 possible neurological side effects/complications of an interscalene block (6 marks). Give one feature that is a hallmark of each complication you list (6 marks)

Complication (6 marks)	**Feature** (6 marks)
1	1 ....
2	2 ....
3	3 ....
4	4 ....
5	5 ....
6	6 ....

Total 20 marks

Question 10

A 25-year-old woman presents to the labour ward in the early stages of labour. She is Para 1 + 0 at 38 weeks' gestation. She has no significant past medical history. She weighs 140kg.

A. Classify obesity using World Health Organization (WHO) definition of BMI (3 marks)

....

B. List 5 risks associated with obesity during pregnancy (5 marks)

1. ....

2. ....

3. ....

4. ....

5. ....

C. List 6 physiological changes that occur in the respiratory system and airway due to obesity? (6 marks)

1. ....

2. ....

3. ....

4. ....

5. ....

6. ....

D. Outline your initial management of this patient on the labour ward (6 marks)

....

....

....

....

....

....

....

....

Total 20 marks

Question 11

A 34 year old man is listed for elective colostomy. He had a complete C6 spinal cord injury 10 years ago.

A. Describe the pathophysiology of autonomic dysreflexia (ADR)? (3 marks)

....

....

....

....

B. What 3 features of a spinal cord injury are usually associated with development of severe ADR? (3 marks)

1. ....

2. ....

3. ....

C. What is the most common precipitant of an episode of ADR in this patient group? (1 mark)

....

D. What are the clinical manifestations which aid recognition of an episode of ADR? (6 marks)

1. ....

2. ....

3. ....

4. ....

5. ....

6. ....

E. List the main anaesthetic techniques which can be considered for elective colostomy formation in this patient (4 marks)

1. ....

2. ....

3. ....

4. ....

F. The patient develops an episode of ADR in HDU 24 hours postoperatively. Briefly describe the management steps (3 marks)

1. ....

2. ....

3. ....

Total 20 marks

Question 12

An 86-year-old female requires preoperative assessment for vitreoretinal surgery.

A. List the patient factors which may require this procedure to be performed under general anaesthesia (3 marks)

1. ....

2. ....

3. ....

B. The patient has no significant medical history. She has not had her blood pressure checked within the last year. She is found to have a blood pressure of 169/94 on a single reading in the preoperative assessment clinic. What actions are appropriate regarding her raised blood pressure? (3 marks)

1. ....

2. ....

3. ....

C. The patient is asking whether general anaesthesia is safe for her.

Briefly describe 3 different modalities which can be used to help inform patients of risk during the consent process? (3 marks)

1. ....

2. ....

3. ....

D. The patient wishes to proceed with the procedure under general anaesthesia and supplemental block performed asleep.

List 4 principles of general anaesthesia for intraocular eye surgery (4 marks)

1. ....

2. ....

3. ....

4. ....

E. Describe a single eye block by completing the following table (3 marks)

Block (1 mark)	Eye position for block (1 mark)	Needle insertion point (1 mark)
....	....	....
....	....	....

F. List 4 of the complications specific to eye blocks? (4 marks)

1. ....

2. ....

3. ....

4. ....

Total 20 marks

Exam 4 **Answers**

Many of the following questions contain more answers than there are marks allocated. This redundancy is intentional and is to ensure that a spread of possible answers by the candidate are recognized. 1 mark is awarded per correct point up to the maximum specified in each subsection.

Question 1

A 67-year-old patient is on the trauma list for emergency surgery for fractured neck of femur. He was fitted with a permanent pacemaker 5 years ago, after suffering blackouts. His pacemaker code is DDI.

A. Describe what each letter of this pacemaker code denotes? (3 marks)

1. Chamber paced (Dual)
2. Chamber sensed (Dual)
3. Response to sensing I or E, inhibitory, or excitatory. (3)

B. This is the patient's ECG on admission. What information about the pacemaker can be deduced from this? (3 marks)

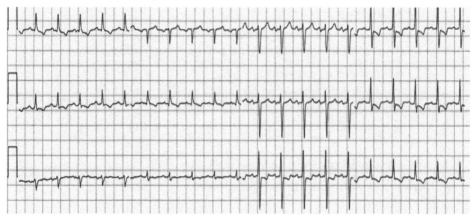

1. There is no evidence of pacemaker activity.
2. This may mean the pacemaker is functioning normally and is inhibited while the intrinsic heart rate remains above threshold

OR

3. It could mean the pacemaker is not working. (3)

C. You decide to change the pacemaker to fixed rate pacing. What pacemaker code denotes fixed rate pacing? (1 mark)

VOO   (1)

D. What is the major concern if this pacemaker is subject to electrical interference? (2 marks)

Electrical interference from other sources may be interpreted by the pacemaker as intrinsic cardiac activity (1 mark) and any pacing will be inhibited (1 mark)   (2)

E. What information do positions 4 and 5 of the pacemaker code denote? (2 marks)

1. Programmability (O = none, R = rate modulation)
2. Antitachycardia functions (0 = none, P = pace, S = shock, D = dual pace and shock)   (2)

F. Describe what each position (1–4) of an implantable defibrillation device code denotes (4 marks)

1. Position 1—shock chamber (O = none, A = atrium, V—ventricle, D = dual)
2. Position 2—chamber where antitachycardia pacing delivered (O = none, A = atrium, V—ventricle, D = dual)
3. Position 3—how tachyarrhythmia is detected (E = electrocardiogram, H = haemodynamically)
4. Position 4 denotes pacemaker capability of the device   (4)

G. How would you advise the theatre team in the safe use of monopolar diathermy? (3 marks)

1. Place diathermy earthing pad away from chest
2. Use diathermy in short bursts rather than for long continuous periods
3. External defibrillator/pacer location known and nearby
4. Have a plan for where to site gel pads should defibrillation be required   (3)

H. State which anaesthetic technique you would use for this patient (1 mark) and why (1 mark)

1. General anaesthesia—better physiological control

OR

2. Regional anaesthesia—real time monitor of effects of cardiovascular changes on patient well-being. Continual cerebral monitoring   (2)

Total 20 marks

Further reading

P Diprose, JM Pierce; Anaesthesia for patients with pacemakers and similar devices. British Journal of Anaesthesia CEPD Reviews, Volume 1, Issue 6, 2001, Pages 166–70.

TV Salukhe, D Dob, R Sutton; Pacemakers and defibrillators: anaesthetic implications, BJA: British Journal of Anaesthesia, Volume 93, Issue 1, July 2004, Pages 95–104.

Question 2

A 4-year-old boy is listed for strabismus surgery as a day case.

A. **List the general** (4 marks) and specific (4 marks) anaesthetic issues.

General considerations (4 marks)

1. Consent from parents
2. Fasting
3. Induction: IV or gas
4. Venous access may be challenging
5. Patient anxiety/lack of cooperation
6. Consider premedication: both topical local anaesthetic to hands and anxiolytic if indicated (4)

Specific to this procedure (4 marks)

1. Brisk oculocardiac reflex
2. Postoperative nausea and vomiting
3. Operation site close to the airway
4. Increased risk of rare muscle problems presenting for the 1st time (e.g. muscular dystrophies)
5. Raised risk of malignant hyperpyrexia in this patient group
6. Unpredictable response to non-depolarizing muscle relaxants (NDMR) (4)

B. **How would you manage profound bradycardia during surgical traction?** (3 marks)

1. Ask the surgeon to stop immediately
2. Ask for senior help
3. Give atropine 20 mcg/kg (estimated weight 16kg = 320mcg atropine)
4. If no response, elevate arm, flush IV, and start cardiac compressions

Note: 1 mark for each, drug dose must be given (3)

C. For each of these 3 common postoperative problems, complete the table with the relevant management strategies (9 marks)

Post-op problem	Management 1 (3 marks)	Management 2 (3 marks)	Management 3 (3 marks)
PONV	Prophylactic antiemetic, e.g. ondansetron 0.15mg/kg +/–dexamethasone 0.15mg/kg Combination increases efficacy (1)	Rescue antiemetic e.g. IV dexamethasone 0.15mg/kg slow IV or droperidol 0.025mg/kg No benefit to repeat ondansetron (1)	Ensure fluid balance and minimize fasting time (mark also given for acupuncture point P6 stimulation) (1)
Pain	Intraoperative paracetamol 15–20mg/kg (1)	Diclofenac 1mg/kg (1)	Local anaesthetic infiltration by surgeon intraoperatively (1)
Recovery room distress	Reunite with parents early to manage distress and anxiety (1)	Treat or exclude pain (1)	Distraction with play therapist (1)

Note: There is no evidence for metoclopramide or prochlorperazine (stemetil) in children and it is not recommended. (9)

Total 20 marks

Further reading

I Barker (ed.), Royal College of Anaesthetists; *Raising the Standard: A Compendium of Audit Recipes* 3rd Edition 2012, Section 9: Paediatrics.

I James; Anaesthesia for paediatric eye surgery, *BJA Education Continuing Education in Anaesthesia, Critical Care and Pain*, Volume 8, Issue 1, 1st February 2008, Pages 5–10.

L Link Tan, G Meakin; Anaesthesia for the uncooperative child, *Continuing Education in Anaesthesia, Critical Care and Pain*, Volume 10, 2010, Pages 48–52.

S Martin, D Baines, H Holtby, AS Carr; *The Association of Paediatrics Anaesthetist of Great Britain and Ireland Guidelines on the Prevention of Postoperative Vomiting in Children* 2016 https://www.apagbi.org.uk/sites/default/files/inline-files/2016%20APA%20POV%20Guideline-2.pdf

POEMS for children UK Charity https://www.poemsforchildren.co.uk

Question 3

A 52-year-old woman is having a right nephrectomy. She has a past medical history of hypertension for which she takes atenolol. Induction and intubation with propofol and rocuronium were straightforward. You transfer her into theatre and administer prophylactic gentamicin. Twenty minutes later, as the abdomen is being prepped her blood pressure drops to 79/32, her heart rate is 132bpm, and her airway pressures increase. You suspect anaphylaxis.

A. **Outline your immediate management** (4 marks)

1. Declare critical incident and call for help
2. Use anaphylaxis emergency box
3. Stop administration of potential causative agent
4. Maintain airway and give 100% oxygen
5. Give epinephrine (adrenaline) 0.5mg IM adrenaline (0.5mls of 1:1,000). Alternately consider intravenous adrenaline which may be titrated to effect in small boluses if familiar with its use (e.g. 0.5–1ml bolus of 1:10,000 and repeat to effect. Consider adrenaline infusion)
6. Rapid infusion of 1–2L of crystalloid

Note: Must have declared incident and used adrenaline for full marks (4)

B. **Outline your secondary management** (3 marks)

1. Chlorpheniramine 10mg IV
2. Hydrocortisone 200mg IV
3. Give salbutamol and or magnesium for bronchospasm/high airway pressures
4. Bloods for mast cell tryptase as per protocols
5. Consider repeat adrenaline/infusion as necessary (3)

C. **The patient's blood pressure remains at 75/42mmHg. You administer a further fluid bolus. What other secondary agents would you consider to treat the refractory hypotension?** (2 marks)

1. Glucagon bolus and infusion to counteract beta-blockade
2. Noradrenaline
3. Vasopressin

Note: Must have glucagon for both marks (2)

D. **In the NAP6 study what are the 3 most common causative agents of perioperative anaphylaxis?** (3 marks)

1. Neuromuscular blocking drugs
2. Antibiotics
3. Chlorhexidine (3)

E. Complete the following table with the different hypersensitivity reactions (8 marks)

TYPE	Description of immune response (4 marks)	Example (4 marks)
1	Immediate response. IgE mediated causing degranulation of mast cells (1)	Anaphylaxis (1)
2	Cytotoxic reactions caused by circulating antibodies (IgG and IgM) reacting with antigens in the presence of complement causing cell lysis (1)	Autoimmune haemolytic anaemia Thrombocytopenia Myasthenia gravis Graves' disease (any 1)
3	Immune complex mediated antibody (IgG) binds to a soluble antigen forming a circulating immune complex. These deposit in blood vessels, kidneys, and joints (1)	Serum sickness Rheumatoid arthritis SLE Post-streptococcus glomerulonephritis (any 1)
4	T-cell mediated Delayed type hypersensitivity (1)	Contact dermatitis Chronic transplant rejection (any 1)

(8)

Total 20 marks

Further reading

National Audit Projects; *Anaesthesia, Surgery and Life-Threatening Allergic Reactions* https://www.nationalauditprojects.org.uk/NAP6

Question 4

A 52-year-old man is ventilated in the ICU. He presented 4 days ago with severe community acquired pneumonia. You now suspect he has ARDS.

A. Detail the current criteria for the diagnosis of ARDS? (8 marks)

1. Berlin Criteria (1)
2. *Timing*—within 1 week of a known clinical insult or new/worsening respiratory symptoms (1)
3. *Chest imaging* (chest X-ray (CXR) or CT)—bilateral opacities not fully explained by effusions, lobar collapse, or nodules (1)

4. *Origin of oedema*—respiratory failure not fully explained by cardiac failure or fluid overload (1)
5. *Oxygenation* (1)
6. Mild—PaO_2/FiO_2 = 26.6–49.9kPa with positive end-expiratory pressure (PEEP) or CPAP> 5cm H_2O (1)
7. Moderate PaO_2/FiO_2 = 13.3kPa—26.6kPa with PEEP or CPAP> 5cm H_2O (1)
8. Severe PaO_2/FiO_2 <13.3kPA with PEEP> 5 cm H_2O (1)   (8)

B. Describe the pathophysiology of ARDS (4 marks)

ARDS is the result of:

1. Release of inflammatory mediators
2. Diffuse alveolar damage
3. Non-cardiogenic pulmonary oedema
4. Surfactant dysfunction
5. Atelectasis
6. Fibrosis   (4)

C. Complete the table to describe each of the 3 phases of ARDS (3 marks)

Phase	Pathophysiological description
Acute/exudative (1 mark)	Hypoxia and reduced pulmonary compliance due to alveolar flooding with protein-rich fluid (1)
Proliferative/subacute (1 mark)	Fibroproliferation and microvascular thrombus formation lead to further reduction in compliance and hypoxaemia (1)
Chronic/fibrotic (1 mark)	Widespread fibrosis and lung remodelling which may be irreversible (1)

(3)

D. What specific strategies can be used in the management of ARDS to optimize ventilation and oxygenation? (3 marks)

1. Target tidal volumes of 6ml/kg
2. Avoiding peak plateau pressures >30kPa
3. Using PEEP and increasing it with increasing oxygen requirements
4. Prone positioning
5. ECMO (Extracorporeal membrane oxygenation)   (3)

Note: Do not accept steroids, statins, inhaled nitric oxide, or high frequency oscillation ventilation or optimization of fluid management

E. **List 2 beneficial effects of the prone position in severe ARDS?** (2 marks)

1. Reduction in V/Q mismatch
2. Increase in the functional residual capacity
3. Recruitment of atelectatic lung   (2)

Note: the PROSEVA trial demonstrated a reduction in 28 day mortality, with a number needed to treat of 6.

Total 20 marks

Further reading

V McCormack, S Tolhurst-Cleaver; Acute respiratory distress syndrome, *BJA Education*, Volume 17, Issue 5, 1 May 2017, Pages 161–165.

Question 5

A patient attends the chronic pain clinic with facial pain. Her GP has told her he thinks she has TN.

A. **Give 5 characteristics of the pain that supports a diagnosis of TN?** (5 marks)

1. Pain: sudden severe lancing electric shock
2. Episodic attacks of variable duration, with complete resolution between
3. Attacks triggered by trivial stimuli including teeth brushing, wind, cotton wool, eating
4. Affects 1 (or possibly 2) divisions of the trigeminal nerve (maxillary > mandibular > ophthalmic)
5. No neurological deficit
6. No other cause for pain
7. Affects females > males 2:1
8. Peak age 50–60   (5)

B. **Give 4 differential diagnoses** (4 marks)

1. Migraine
2. Hemi-facial neuralgia or facial cephalgia
3. Dental pain
4. Temporomandibular joint disorder
5. Tumours—acoustic neuroma or meningioma
6. Tension headache   (4)

C. **What other conditions is TN associated with?** (3 marks)

1. Multiple sclerosis
2. Hypertension
3. Previous CVA (3)

D. **What drugs would you use to treat TN?** (3 marks)

1. Carbamazepine (mark only given if this is given as first line/first choice of treatment)
2. Gabapentin OR pregabalin
3. Amitriptyline OR nortriptyline
4. Duloxetine
5. Lamotrigine (3)

E. **What non-pharmacological treatments are available for TN?** (3 marks)

1. Percutaneous procedures that ablate the nerve, its ganglion, or pathway
   - Glycerol neurolysis at Gasserian ganglion (chemical neurolysis)
   - Radiofrequency lesioning of Gasserian ganglion (heat neurolysis, known as DREZ)
   - Balloon compression (pressure neurolysis)
2. Microvascular decompression
3. Stereotactic neurosurgery: radiation to the trigeminal ganglion (3)

F. **If left untreated, what is the natural prognosis of the condition?** (1 mark)

Worsening over time. This pain is also known as the suicide pain (1)

G. **What is the incidence of TN in the UK? Please select your answer** (1 mark)

1 in 10,000 (1)

Total 20 marks

Further reading

NHS Health Website https://www.nhs.uk/conditions/trigeminal-neuralgia/treatment/
NICE Clinical Knowledge Summaries; Trigeminal neuralgia January 2018 https://cks.nice.org.uk/
  trigeminal-neuralgia#!scenario

Note: Carbamazepine will treat 80–90% of cases of TN. If not successful the diagnosis should be revisited. Interventional options are much higher risk and should only be considered when drug therapy has failed or is intolerable, particularly in younger patients. A large part of management is avoiding triggers such as cold, eating on the affected side, hair touching the face, etc.

Question 6

A 61-year-old woman with endometrial cancer is listed for total abdominal hysterectomy and bi-lateral salpingo-ophorectomy with pelvic lymphadenectomy. Her medical history is type 2 diabetes mellitus and asthma. Her medication is metformin, gliclazide, and salbutamol. She is a long-term smoker. Her BMI is 48kg/m^2.

A. **What class of obesity is this patient in?** (1 mark)

1. BMI >40 is obese 3 according to WHO classification of obesity
2. Also considered as morbid obesity in other classifications (1)

B. **Briefly describe the specific preoperative concerns which must be considered in this patient?** (5 marks)

1. Adequacy of diabetic control—HbA1c
2. Airway assessment for increased risk of difficult/failed intubation
3. Distribution of fat—higher perioperative risk in central > peripheral
4. Screening for obstructive sleep apnoea, e.g. STOP-BANG or Epworth. Concern if bicarbonate >28
5. Consider spirometry—Probable restrictive defect due to obesity. Wheeze in the obese may be due to premature airway closure rather than asthma. Lack of reversibility with bronchodilator therapy may help differentiate
6. Evaluation for associated comorbidity such as ischaemic heart disease, including functional capacity, hypertension
7. Screening for risk of venous thromboembolism
8. Smoking cessation advice
9. Presence of iron deficiency anaemia associated with vaginal bleeding
10. Stratification of risk group and discussion with patient (5)

C. **Define the following terms considered when administering anaesthetic drugs to obese patients** (4 marks)

Total body weight (TBW) (1 mark)	The actual weight of the patient
Ideal body weight (IBW) (1 mark)	What the patient should weigh with a normal ratio of lean mass to fat mass. Varies with age and is usually calculated as a function of height and sex
Lean body weight (LBW) (1 mark)	The patient's weight excluding fat
Adjusted body weight (ABW) (1 mark)	Obese individuals have increased lean body mass and an increased volume of distribution for drugs. It is calculated by adding 40% of the excess weight to the IBW

(4)

D. **What are the principles of delivering safe general anaesthesia for this patient assuming risk of sleep disordered breathing?** (5 marks)

1. Avoidance of preoperative sedatives if possible
2. Use of short acting agents
3. Use of depth of anaesthesia monitoring techniques to limit anaesthesia load
4. Use of neuromuscular monitoring to maintain a level of block compatible with surgery and to ensure complete reversal of block before waking the patient
5. Maximal use of local anaesthetic and multimodal opioid-sparing analgesia regime
6. Maintaining a head–up position during recovery
7. Postoperatively—additional time in recovery/monitoring of oxygen saturations until fully mobile postoperatively/consider level 2 (HDU) care
8. Early mobilization/extended prophylaxis (5)

E. **What local anaesthesia based analgesic options may be considered for this case?** (4 marks)

1. Spinal anaesthesia with intrathecal opioid (also consider clonidine)
2. Epidural analgesia, although may reduce postoperative mobility
3. Bilateral transversus abdominus plane (TAP) blocks
4. Intravenous lidocaine infusion
5. Wound catheter local anaesthesia infusion
6. Local infiltration of wound (4)

F. **What anatomical landmark indicates an ideal ramped position before induction of general anaesthesia?** (1 mark)

The tragus of the ear should be level with the sternum (1)

Total 20 marks

Further reading

M Morosan, P Popham; Anaesthesia for gynaecological oncological surgery, *Continuing Education in Anaesthesia, Critical Care & Pain*, Volume 14, Issue 2, 2014, Pages 63–68.

A Munro, A Sjaus, RB George; Anesthesia and analgesia for gynaecological surgery, *Current Opinion in Anesthesiology*, Volume 31, Issue 3, 2018, Pages 274–279.

CE Nightingale, MP Margarson, E Shearer; Peri-operative management of the obese surgical patient 2015, *Anaesthesia*, Volume 20, 2015, Pages 859–876.

Question 7

A. **Please detail the 5 levels of the evidence hierarchy** (5 marks)

1. Level 1 systematic review of RCTs

2. Level 2 single RCT
3. Level 3 observational studies
4. Level 4 case series
5. Level 5 case report (5)

B. **Give 4 types of bias you must be aware of, and state how can they be avoided when carrying out research?** (8 marks)

1. Publication bias: more positive than negative results reach publication. Record all studies including those not published
2. Language bias: more papers in English get published. Some non-English papers are amenable to web based translation services
3. Inference bias: the conclusion is not actually supported by result. Keep the question specific and the answer streamlined. Answer only the question asked
4. Selection bias: the group from which the study subjects recruited should be appropriate. Must be random, avoid volunteers if possible
5. Allocation bias: must be random with researcher and clinician unaware (blinded). You cannot put a patient in a group for the treatment you want them to have or treatment you think they will benefit from
6. Measurement bias: an inaccurate method is being used. Is it subject to expectations of a person measuring it? Patients often want to please by providing an anticipated or correct result. Try to use objective measurement where possible

Note: 4 types × 2 marks each (8)

C. **How can results be misleading despite a double blind RCT?** (2 marks)

1. Highlights effects, not side effects
2. Does not account for people who withdraw early, and why they do so. Were side effects intolerable? Did the drug not work? Were they cured? Did they die?
3. The group who withdrew from the study may be inherently different to the group who completed the study. Must follow up dropouts
4. The results may not be transferable to a different patient population or subgroup (2)

D. **What aspects should you pay particular attention to when appraising a paper?** (5 marks)

1. How was it funded, any sponsorship or conflict of interest?
2. Blinding or no blinding? Was it obvious to the clinicians?
3. Does the conclusion relate to the original hypothesis?
4. Which databases were searched?
5. Are the results the primary outcome or derived variables?
6. Have the correct statistical tests been applied?
7. How were participants selected?
8. Attrition rate. Enrolled numbers vs. number used in outcome results (5)

Total 20 marks

Further reading

G Mitchell; An evidence based resource for pain relief, *BMJ Evidence-Based Medicine*, Volume 6, 2001, Page 136.
P Wiffen, A Moore; Pain leads the way: the development of evidence-based medicine for pain relief.
  International Journal of Clinical Pharmacology & Therapeutics, Volume 54, Issue 7, 2016, Pages 505–513.

Question 8

You anaesthetise a 19-year-old woman for bimaxillary surgery. She has no significant past medical or drug history.

A. **What specifically is bimaxillary surgery?** (1 mark)

It is maxillofacial surgery involving movement in the relationship of both the mandible and maxilla (1)

B. **What are the common indications for this surgery which are relevant to the anaesthetist?** (2 marks)

1. Cosmetic correction of dental malocclusion
2. Correction of deformity/function related to congenital head and neck conditions
3. Severe obstructive sleep apnoea when conservative measures have failed (2)

C. **What are the main airway considerations for this case?** (3 marks)

1. Potential limited mouth opening which may not improve with anaesthesia
2. Possible difficult laryngoscopy in severe malocclusion with consideration of awake fibreoptic intubation
3. Usually mandates nasal intubation to allow intraoperative assessment of dental occlusion
4. Shared airway surgery, risk of endotracheal tube damage or dislodgement intraoperatively (3)

D. **Following successful intubation you insert a throat pack.**

Describe 5 steps that are taken to ensure the throat pack is not retained in error following completion of surgery and anaesthesia? (5 marks)

1. Discussion of intention to use a throat pack during the theatre safety brief
2. Throat packs are routinely included in swab counts
3. Label or mark the patient as having a throat pack *in situ* on either their head or, exceptionally, on another visible part of their body with an adherent sticker or marker
4. Attach the pack securely to the artificial airway
5. Leave part of the pack protruding
6. Document throat pack insertion and removal on the anaesthetic record
7. Throat pack inclusion on theatre checklists (5)

E. What techniques can be used to minimize bleeding during this operation? (2 marks)

1. Head up position
2. No restriction to venous drainage
3. Anaesthetic technique which promotes avoidance/blunting of hypertensive surges
4. Infiltration of local anaesthetic and adrenaline into the operation site   (2)

F. The patient has intramedullary fixation (IMF) with elastics in place at cessation of surgery. What measures are taken to ensure airway safety during emergence from anaesthesia and in the early postoperative period for this situation? (7 marks)

	Airway safety measures
Emergence (4 marks)	1. Airway suctioned under direct vision 2. Excellent upper airway haemostasis 3. Smooth emergence and avoidance of coughing facilitated by remifentanil 4. Partial withdrawal of nasal tracheal tube to function as a nasal airway 5. Continued presence of surgeon in theatre during emergence
Postoperative (3 marks)	1. Vigilance for bleeding/swelling/haematoma formation 2. Bedside availability of scissors to cut elastics 3. Use of antiemetics/avoidance of PONV 4. Monitoring on specialist maxillofacial ward postoperatively

(7)

Total 20 marks

Further reading

JI Beck, KD Johnston; Anaesthesia for cosmetic and functional maxillofacial surgery, *Continuing Education in Anaesthesia Critical Care & Pain*, Volume 14, Issue 1, 2014, Pages 38–42.

NHS Improvement; *Recommendations from National Patient Safety Agency Alerts That Remain Relevant to the Never Events List* 2018 https://improvement.nhs.uk/documents/2267/Recommendations_from_NPSA_alerts_that_remain_relevant_to_NEs_FINAL.pdf

L Kersanx, L Kersan, U Ratnasabapathy; Anaesthesia for maxillofacial surgery, *Anaesthesia and Intensive Care Medicine*, Volume 18, Issue 9, 2017, Pages 442–446.

Question 9

You assess a 24-year-old rugby player for repair of rotator cuff in his right shoulder. He weighs 110kg and is 185cm tall. He is right-handed.

A. Name 4 nerves that need to be blocked to provide analgesia for rotator cuff repair (4 marks)

1. supraclavicular nerve
2. axillary nerve

3. supra scapular nerve
4. dorsal scapular nerves
5. lateral pectoral nerve
6. plus variable small contributions from
    1. medial cutaneous nerve
    2. musculocutaneous nerve
    3. intercostobrachial nerve

(4)

B. **What are the benefits of the interscalene approach to the brachial plexus in this case?** (4 marks)

1. Covers most of the nerves required for proximal upper limb analgesia
2. Reliable
3. Single injection
4. Superficial injection

(4)

C. Complete the table by listing 6 possible neurological side effects/complications of an interscalene block? (6 marks)

Give one feature that is a hallmark of each complication you list (6 marks)

Complication (6 marks)	**Feature** (6 marks)
1. Phrenic nerve block	1. Respiratory difficulty especially when taking deep breaths
2. Stellate ganglion block	2. Horner's syndrome, ipsilateral meiosis, ptosis, enophthalmos
3. Vagus nerve block	3. Hiccoughs
4. Unilateral recurrent laryngeal nerve block	4. Hoarseness, stridor, loss, or change in voice. Vocal cord adduction
5. Total spinal vertebral artery injection	5. Arrythmia, seizure, loss of consciousness
6. Epidural injection	6. Inadequate block, bilateral spread with a high sensory/motor level
7. Neuropraxia	7. Temporary loss of motor function in part of the upper limb after the block has worn off

Complication (6 marks)	Feature (6 marks)
8. Brachial plexus damage	8. Non-resolving symptoms after the block has worn off
9. Cervical cord damage	9. Unilateral signs, sensory or motor, including hemiplegia

Total 20 marks

Further reading

CL Beecroft, DM Coventry; Anaesthesia for shoulder surgery, *Continuing Education in Anaesthesia Critical Care & Pain*, Volume 8, Issue 6, December 2008, Pages 193–198.

Question 10

A 25-year-old woman presents to the labour ward in the early stages of labour. She is Para 1 + 0 at 38 weeks' gestation. She has no significant past medical history. She weighs 140kg.

A. Classify obesity using the WHO definition of BMI (3 marks)

BMI = weight(kg)/height (m) squared (1 mark)

Mild Obesity or class 1 obesity 30–34.9

Moderate obesity or class 2 obesity 35–39.9

Severe or morbid obesity or class 3 obesity >40

(1 mark for categories mild/moderate/severe or 1–3 and final 1 mark for correct ranges)　　(3)

B. List 5 risks associated with obesity during pregnancy (5 marks)

Increased risk of:

1. miscarriage and stillbirth
2. foetal abnormality
3. PIH/pre-eclampsia
4. gestational diabetes
5. postpartum haemorrhage
6. thromboembolic event
7. wound infection
8. requiring induction and or augmentation of labour
9. instrumental delivery and caesarean section　　(5)

C. List 6 physiological changes that may occur in the respiratory system due to obesity?
(6 marks)

1. Higher incidence of difficult airway and intubation
2. Higher incidence of regurgitation and aspiration
3. Reduced functional residual capacity (FRC) and increased oxygen consumption (faster desaturation)
4. Reduced closing capacity
5. Restrictive respiratory pattern due to the additional weight on the thorax and restriction of diaphragm movement leading to impaired diaphragm function
6. Poor lung compliance
7. Increased pulmonary resistance
8. Higher incidence of obstructive sleep apnoea (OSA)
9. Increased work of breathing
10. Increased V:Q mismatch
11. Obese hypoventilation syndrome (Pickwickian syndrome)   (6)

D. Outline your initial management of this patient on the labour ward (6 marks)

1. Full history and examination including airway assessment, examination of lumbar spine, and anaesthetic history
2. Discuss risks and benefits of analgesic options
3. Recommend early epidural
4. Ensure epidural is working adequately in labour
5. Inform senior anaesthetic, obstetric, and midwifery staff of high risk patient to establish multidisciplinary plan
6. Early IV access
7. Antacid prophylaxis
8. Clear oral fluids during labour only   (6)

Total 20 marks

Further reading

Royal College of Obstetricians and Gynaecologists; *CMACE/RCOG Joint Guideline—Management of Women with Obesity in Pregnancy* March 2010 https://www.rcog.org.uk/globalassets/documents/guidelines/cmacercogjoi ntguidelinemanagementwomenobesitypregnancya.pdf

Question 11

A 34-year-old man is listed for elective colostomy. He had a complete C6 spinal cord injury 10 years ago.

A. Describe the pathophysiology of autonomic dysreflexia (ADR) (3 marks)

1. It is a disorganized spinal sympathetic response to stimuli below the level of the lesion. Spinal circuits below the lesion are established and result in exaggerated responses
2. Sympathetic activation causes massive vasoconstriction and hypertension
3. Intact baroreceptors sense the hypertension causing a reflex bradycardia mediated by the intact Vagus nerve (CN X)
4. Descending inhibitory pathways are not transmitted due to the discontinuous cord (3)

B. **What 3 features of a spinal cord injury are usually associated with development of severe ADR?** (3 marks)

1. Complete spinal cord injury is more severe than incomplete injury
2. More severe with higher spinal cord lesions (e.g. above T6 often quoted)
3. More prevalent with higher spinal cord lesions
4. Most commonly observed in the chronic stage i.e. > 1 year after spinal cord injury (3)

C. **What is the most common precipitant of an episode of ADR in this patient group?** (1 mark)

1. Bladder or bowel distension (1)

D. **What are the clinical manifestations which aid recognition of an episode of ADR?** (6 marks)

1. Increased BP of at least 20%
2. Headache
3. Flushing
4. Sweating
5. Chills
6. Nasal congestion
7. Piloerection
8. Pallor
9. Severe sequelae in late presentation—seizures, intracranial haemorrhage, myocardial ischaemia, arrhythmias, pulmonary oedema (6)

E. **List the main anaesthetic techniques which can be considered for elective colostomy formation in this patient** (4 marks)

1. No anaesthesia, anaesthetist on standby
2. General anaesthesia
3. Neuraxial technique—spinal or epidural
4. Combined general and neuraxial technique (4)

F. **The patient develops an episode of ADR in HDU 24 hours postoperatively.**

Briefly describe the management steps (3 marks)

1. Sit the patient up, remove support stockings
2. Exclude bladder/bowel distension—check catheter and perform abdominal exam

3. 1st line pharmacological management: consider sublingual glyceryl trinitrate (GTN), sublingual nifedipine

4. 2nd line pharmacological management: consider intravenous therapy such as glyceryl trinitrate, hydralazine, diazoxide, phentolamine, or magnesium (3)

Total 20 marks

Further reading

A Petsas, J Drake; Perioperative management for patients with a spinal cord injury, *BJA Education*, Volume 15, Issue 3, 2015, Pages 123–130.

Question 12

An 86-year-old female requires preoperative assessment for vitreoretinal surgery.

A. **List the patient factors which may require this procedure to be performed under general anaesthesia** (3 marks)

1. Longer duration more likely in vitreoretinal surgery
2. Inability to lie flat due to severe comorbidity (heart failure, severe COPD)
3. Unable to cooperate (e.g. cognitive dysfunction)
4. Refusal of awake surgery
5. Movement disorder (3)

B. **The patient has no significant medical history. She has not had her blood pressure checked within the last year. She is found to have a blood pressure of 169/94 on a single reading in the preoperative assessment clinic.**

   What actions are appropriate regarding her raised blood pressure? (3 marks)

1. Measure blood pressure 3 times and choose lowest numbers
2. Proceed to elective surgery without delay as per AAGBI/BHS guidelines if BP <180/110
3. Screen for signs of hypertension related end organ damage e.g. ECG for LVH, U&E for raised creatinine
4. Inform GP of findings
5. No need for repeated or home blood pressure monitoring by the preoperative assessment clinic (3)

C. **The patient is asking whether general anaesthesia is safe for her.**

   Briefly describe 3 different modalities which can be used to help inform patients of risk during the consent process? (3 marks)

1. Face to face discussion
2. Analogy e.g. 1 in a street, 1 in a town, 1 in a city
3. Infographics e.g. Royal College of Anaesthetists' resources

4. Written leaflet to take away

5. Signposting to online resources (3)

D. The patient wishes to proceed with the procedure under general anaesthesia and supplemental block performed asleep.

List 4 principles of general anaesthesia for intraocular eye surgery (4 marks)

1. Minimize increases in intraocular pressure/volume

2. Use of antimuscarinic (e.g. atropine, glycopyrrolate) may be considered as prophylaxis against oculocardiac reflex

3. Controlled ventilation to control CO_2

4. Avoid nitrous oxide in vitreoretinal surgery

5. Supplementary analgesia provided ideally with local anaesthesia block

6. Avoidance of coughing/movement intraoperatively e.g. maintain muscle paralysis throughout

7. Smooth emergence without coughing e.g. use of flexible laryngeal mask airway (LMA) in preference to endotracheal intubation if appropriate

8. Routine use of antiemetics (4)

E. Describe a single eye block by completing the following table (3 marks)

Block (1 mark)	Eye position for block (1 mark)	Needle insertion point (1 mark)
1. Sub-tenon injection	1. Eye looks up and out	1. Inferonasal, 5–10mm from the limbus
2. Peribulbar injection	2. Eye neutral in position	2. Inferotemporal corner
3. Retrobulbar injection	3. Eye in neutral position	3. Junction of lateral 1/3 and medial 2/3 of lower orbital ridge

Note: Subtenon block is by far the most common. Retrobulbar eye block is not now recommended because of complication rates but is included for completeness and historical reasons. (3)

F. List 4 of the complications specific to eye blocks? (4 marks)

1. Chemosis (swollen conjunctiva)

2. Conjunctival haematoma

3. Globe perforation

4. Vascular injection

5. Retro-orbital vascular damage and haemorrhage

6. Optic nerve damage/altered acuity/sight loss

7. Brain-stem anaesthesia (4)

Total 20 marks

Further reading

R Anker, N Kaur; Regional anaesthesia for ophthalmic surgery, *BJA Education*, Volume 17, Issue 7, 2017, Pages 221–227.

M Crowther, K van der Spuy, F Roodt, et al.; The relationship between pre-operative hypertension and intra-operative haemodynamic changes known to be associated with postoperative morbidity, *Anaesthesia*, Volume 73, 2018, Pages 812–818.

A Hartle, T McCormack, J Carlisle, et al.; The measurement of adult blood pressure and management of hypertension before elective surgery, *Anaesthesia*, Volume 71, 2016, Pages 326–337.

Exam 5 **Questions**

Exam 5 contains 12 selected Constructed Response Questions (CRQs) balanced across the intermediate curriculum, reflecting the Final Examination of the Diploma of Fellowship of the Royal College of Anaesthetists (FRCA) exam. We recommend attempting these questions under exam conditions. Please limit/contain your answer to/within the dotted lines given for each question.

Question 1

A 69-year-old man presents following an episode of amaurosis fugax. His investigations have identified an 80% stenosis of his left carotid artery. You see him in the preoperative period.

A. What is the optimal medical management of this clinical picture? (4 marks)

....

....

....

....

B. Following a multidisciplinary team discussion, he is to have a left carotid endarterectomy. List the advantages and disadvantages of regional anaesthesia for this operation (6 marks)

Advantages (3 marks)	Disadvantages (3 marks)

C. You are going to perform deep and superficial cervical plexus blocks as part of your anaesthetic management. Outline the relevant anatomy of the cervical plexus for the blocks (2 marks)

D. You intend to perform a deep cervical plexus block. The patient has given full informed consent for the procedure. You have established intravenous access, full Association of Anaesthetists of Great Britain and Ireland (AAGBI) monitoring and have a trained assistant. Patient is awake and you use an aseptic technique.

Describe how you would position the patient and identify points for injection (4 marks)

E. Now you have confirmed the appropriate anatomy, detail how you would complete the block and inject the local anaesthetic (4 marks)

Total 20 marks

Question 2

A 74-year-old woman presents to the emergency department with a 24-hour history of severe abdominal pain and signs of septic shock. She has a history of transient ischaemic attack. Her drug history is clopidogrel. Erect chest X-ray shows a pneumoperitoneum. The surgeons request anaesthetic review pending urgent laparotomy.

A. What modifiable, organizational factors contribute to poor outcomes in patients requiring emergency laparotomy? (2 marks)

1. ....

2. ....

B. Briefly describe 5 recommended standards of care for a high-risk patient from the third National Emergency Laparotomy Audit (NELA) report (5 marks)

1. ....

2. ....

3. ....

4. ....

5. ....

C. List 4 commonly quoted risk calculators used for general surgery patients undergoing emergency laparotomy (4 marks)

1. ....

2. ....

3. ....

4. ....

D. On further assessment, the patient has a prominent history of side effects due to high dose systemic opioids

What measures, additional to simple analgesics, can be considered to facilitate an opioid sparing anaesthetic technique in this patient? (4 marks)

1. ....

2. ....

3. ....

4. ....

E. What intraoperative targets are recommended during management of an emergency laparotomy patient with signs of septic shock? (5 marks)

System	Goals
Cardiovascular (2 marks)	1. .... 2. ....
Respiratory (3 marks)	1. .... 2. .... 3. ....

Total 20 marks

Question 3

A 79-year-old life-long smoker attends for preoperative assessment, prior to right pneumonectomy.

A. List the absolute (3 marks) and relative (2 marks) indications for placement of a double lumen tube in anaesthesia and critical care.

Absolute

Relative

B. List methods of preoperative respiratory assessment you may use in an adult to assess their suitability for pneumonectomy. Give threshold values where required (5 marks)

C. How would you manage hypoxaemia during one-lung anaesthesia? (8 marks)

1. ....

2. ....

3. ....

4. ....

5. ....

6. ....

7. ....

8. ....

D. What is ventilation-perfusion coupling? What does it achieve? (2 marks)

....

....

Total marks 20

Question 4

A. List 4 risk factors for pre-eclampsia (4 marks)

1. ....

2. ....

3. ....

4. ....

B. List criteria used in the diagnosis of mild pre-eclampsia (3 marks)

1. ....

2. ....

3. ....

C. List 3 drugs and their doses you would use to treat hypertension, and *in the order* you would use them (3 marks)

Antihypertensive choice	Drug	Initial dose and route	Maintenance
1st (1 mark)			
2nd (1 mark)			
3rd (1 mark)			

D. Give 2 further signs or symptoms that define pre-eclampsia as being severe (2 marks)

1. ....

2. ....

E. Give details of the magnesium administration regimen used in severe pre-eclampsia (2 marks)

....

....

F. List 3 signs or symptoms of magnesium toxicity (3 marks)

1. ....

2. ....

3. ....

G. How should magnesium toxicity be managed? (3 marks)

....

....

....

Total 20 marks

Question 5

A 39-year-old man is scheduled for the excision of a medulloblastoma from his posterior cranial fossa. He is to be in the sitting position for his surgery.

A. List 3 contraindications to the sitting position (3 marks)

1. ....

2. ....

3. ....

B. What are the complications associated with surgery in the sitting position? (3 marks)

....

....

....

C. List 2 ways in which the risk of venous air embolism can be minimized (2 marks)

1. ....

2. ....

D. Complete this table with the clinical features of venous air embolism (8 marks)

Cardiovascular (4 marks)	
	....
	....
	....
	....
Respiratory (3 marks)	....
	....
	....
CNS (1 mark)	....

E. List 4 specific monitors that can be used to detect venous air embolism during anaesthesia (4 marks)

1. ....

2. ....

3. ....

4. ....

Total 20 marks

Question 6

A 49-year-old woman requires elective total thyroidectomy. She has a history of hyperthyroidism and Graves' disease. Her drug history includes carbimazole and propranolol.

A. Give 2 clinical features which are specific to Graves' disease (2 marks)

1. ....

2. ....

B. List 4 preoperative signs specific to goitre which may indicate potential airway difficulty during induction of anaesthesia (4 marks)

1. ....

2. ....

3. ....

4. ....

C. What clinical signs of hyperthyroidism can be detected at the bedside? (4 marks)

System	Signs
CNS (1 marks)	1. ....
CVS (2 marks)	1. .... 2. ....
General (1 mark)	1. ....

D. What are the biochemical indicators of hyperthyroid disease? (1 mark)

....

....

E. During surgery the patient becomes acutely unwell. You suspect thyroid storm. List 4 of the classical presenting features of thyroid storm (4 marks)

1. ....

2. ....

3. ....

4. ....

F. Explain the importance of checking serum calcium postoperatively following total thyroid surgery (1 mark)

....

....

G. Name the clinical signs which may be elicited on examination in this situation and describe their associated examination findings (4 marks)

Clinical sign (2 marks)	Examination findings (2 marks)
....	....
....	....

Total 20 marks

Question 7

A 6-year-old child presents with a dental abscess requiring surgery. She suffers from Down's syndrome. She has mild developmental delay and cannot cooperate with preoperative assessment.

A. Define Down's syndrome (2 marks)

....

....

B. List the airway issues relevant to the anaesthetic management of this particular child (6 marks)

1. ....

2. ....

3. ....

4. ....

5. ....

6. ....

C. Give 2 options for induction of anaesthesia (1 mark)

....

....

D. Complete the table evaluating the risks and benefits of each method (8 marks)

Technique	Pros (4 marks)	Cons (4 marks)
IV induction/ RSI	1. .... 2. .... 3. .... (2)	1. .... 2. .... 3. .... (2)
Gas induction	1. .... 2. .... 3. .... (2)	1. .... 2. .... 3. .... (2)

E. Give 3 postoperative considerations (3 marks)

1. ....

2. ....

3. ....

Total 20 marks

Question 8

A 29-year-old woman is ventilated in intensive care unit (ICU). She was admitted 48 hours ago with community acquired pneumonia. She has a history of anorexia nervosa and depression. She weighs 46kg.

A. What are the effects of malnutrition in the critical care patient? (3 marks)

....

....

....

....

B. You commence enteral feeding via the nasogastric route. What are the risk factors for developing refeeding syndrome in critical care patients? (4 marks)

1. ....

2. ....

3. ....

4. ....

C. Describe the metabolic changes that occur in refeeding syndrome? (3 marks)

....

....

....

....

D. List 6 clinical features of refeeding syndrome? (6 marks)

....

....

....

....

....

....

E. What are the National Institute for Health and Care (NICE) recommendations for nutrition in patients at high risk of developing refeeding syndrome? (4 marks)

Total 20 marks

Question 9

A 61-year-old unknown male is admitted to the intensive care unit with deteriorating conscious level. He is intubated and ventilated. The neurology team have recommended further investigation with an MRI scan of the head.

A. What logistical challenges are faced by the anaesthetist taking an intensive care patient for MRI scan? (5 marks)

1.

2.

3.

4.

5.

B. What magnetic field strengths are typically used in an MRI scanner? (1 mark)

C. What is the fringe field (1 mark) and its significance? (2 marks)

....

....

....

D. The patient has now been transferred to the anaesthetic room outside the MRI scanner.

Briefly describe 5 of the steps which should be performed to ensure the patient remains safe before entering the magnetic field (5 marks)

1. ....

2. ....

3. ....

4. ....

5. ....

E. Outline the potential MRI-specific hazards to this patient inside the scanning room (5 marks)

1. ....

2. ....

3. ....

4. ....

5. ....

F. Describe the problem encountered following spontaneous or emergency shutdown of the magnetic field (1 mark)

....

....

Total 20 marks

Question 10

A 9-year-old child requires anaesthesia for appendicectomy. He has been vomiting and you plan a rapid sequence induction.

A. What is the physiological basis for preoxygenation prior to anaesthesia? (2 marks)

B. What are the advantages and disadvantages of preoxygenating a child in this scenario? (4 marks)

Advantages (2 marks)	Disadvantages (2 marks)

C. How you would assess the efficacy of preoxygenation? (3 marks)

D. Label the 4 cartilaginous structures within the larynx indicated on the diagram (4 marks)

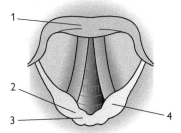

Reproduced from *Training in Anaesthesia*, Catherine Spoors and Kevin Kiff, Figure 6.10. Copyright Oxford University Press, 2011. Reproduced with permission of the Licensor through PLSclear.

1. ....

2. ....

3. ....

4. ....

E. Name the remaining 2 unpaired cartilages of the larynx (2 marks)

1. ....

2. ....

F. At the end of the operation you extubate the child. The abdomen is moving but no airflow is detected at the mouth. You diagnose laryngospasm.

Outline the pathophysiology of laryngospasm (5 marks)

....

....

....

....

....

....

Question 11

You are asked to urgently assess a 2-year-old boy in the emergency department who has stridor of acute onset over 2–3 hours. He is sitting upright with suprasternal and subcostal recession. He has no medical history.

A. What is the definition of stridor? (2 marks)

....

....

B. Why are paediatric airways more prone to stridor than adults? (2 marks)

1. ....

2. ....

C. List discriminating features of the differential diagnoses provided (13 marks)

Croup (3 marks)	1. ....
	2. ....
	3. ....
Epiglottitis (3 marks)	1. ....
	2. ....
	3. ....
Anaphylaxis (2 marks)	1. ....
	2. ....

Inhaled foreign body (2 marks)	1.
	2.
Bacterial tracheitis (3 marks)	1.
	2.
	3.

D. Briefly describe 3 main principles in the management of croup (3 marks)

1.

2.

3.

Total 20 marks

Question 12

A 76-year-old lady presents with an infected hip replacement. She is scheduled for a revision hip replacement. You intend to use cell salvage as part of your perioperative management.

A. Describe the process of cell salvage from surgical site to reinfusion of red cells to the patient (5 marks)

B. What specific considerations are there for cell salvage in this particular patient? (3 marks)

C. You also intend to use thromboelastography (TEG) as part of your management.

What is TEG? (2 marks)

D. What are the limitations of TEG? (4 marks)

E. Identify and describe the clinical significance of the following parameters obtained from a TEG in the following table (6 marks)

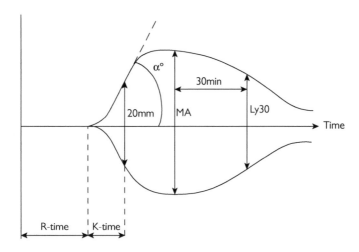

Reproduced from *SAQs for the Final FRCA,* Shorthouse J et al., Figure 3. Copyright Oxford University Press, 2011. Reproduced with permission of the Licensor through PLSclear.

	Name	Description
R (2 marks)		
α angle (2 marks)		
MA (2 marks)		

Total 20 marks

Exam 5 **Answers**

Many of the following questions contain more answers than there are marks allocated. This redundancy is intentional and is to ensure that a spread of possible answers by the candidate are recognized. 1 mark is awarded per correct point up to the maximum specified in each subsection.

Question 1

A 69-year-old man presents following an episode of amaurosis fugax. His investigations have identified an 80% stenosis of his left carotid artery. You see him in the preoperative period.

A. What is the optimal medical management of this clinical picture? (4 marks)

1. Antiplatelet therapy
2. Treatment of hypertension
3. Statin and diet control to lower cholesterol
4. Smoking cessation advice
5. Reduction in alcohol consumption (4)

B. Following a multidisciplinary team discussion, he is to have a left carotid endarterectomy.

List the advantages and disadvantages of regional anaesthesia for this operation (6 marks)

Advantages (3 marks)	**Disadvantages** (3 marks)
1. Allows real time neurological monitoring 2. Avoids risks of airway intervention 3. Decreased shunt rate 4. Allows arterial closure at 'normal' BP with potential reduction in the risk of post-op haematoma (3)	1. Risks from performing block 2. Requires still, co-operative patient. 3. Restricted access to airway 4. Risks of conversion to general anaesthetic (GA) if complications arise 5. Patient stress or pain may increase the risk of myocardial ischaemia (3)

(6)

C. You are going to perform deep and superficial cervical plexus blocks as part of your anaesthetic management.

Outline the relevant anatomy and relations of the cervical plexus for the blocks (2 marks)

1. The plexus sits on the anterior surface of the 4 upper cervical vertebrae
2. It is inferior to the sternocleidomastoid muscle
3. The cervical plexus is formed from the anterior divisions of the 4 upper cervical nerves C1–C4 (2)

Note: The first cervical root is primarily motor and not of major concern for regional anaesthesia. It is the anterior rami of C2–C4 that are important.

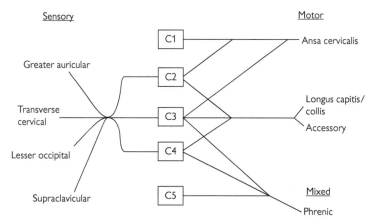

Reproduced from *SAQs for the Final FRCA*, Shorthouse J et al., Figure 10. Copyright Oxford University Press, 2011. Reproduced with permission of the Licensor through PLSclear.

D. You intend to perform a deep cervical plexus block. The patient has given full informed consent for the procedure. You have established intravenous access, full AAGBI monitoring, and have a trained assistant. The patient is awake and you use an aseptic technique.

Describe how you would position the patient and identify points for injection (4 marks)

1. Patient supine with head turned to opposite side (1)
2. Two landmarks marked: Mastoid process (C1) and Chassaignac's tubercle (transverse process of C6)
3. Line drawn between these 2 points over the posterior border of sternocleidomastoid
4. Equidistant marks are made to identify C2, C3, and C4 and block can be done with 3 injections at C2, C3, and C4 or a single injection at C3 or C4 (4)

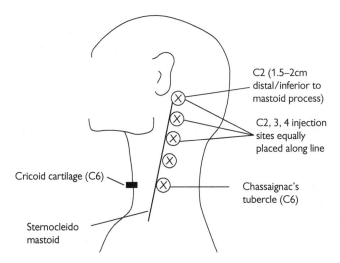

C2 (1.5–2cm distal/inferior to mastoid process)

C2, 3, 4 injection sites equally placed along line

Cricoid cartilage (C6)

Chassaignac's tubercle (C6)

Sternocleido mastoid

E. **Now you have confirmed the appropriate anatomy, detail how you would complete the block and inject the local anaesthetic** (4 marks)

1. STOP BEFORE YOU BLOCK
2. Subcutaneous local anaesthetic (1% lidocaine) administration along the posterior border of sternocleidomastoid
3. Insert short-bevelled 22G needle until contact with transverse process at C2, C3, and C4 then withdraw 1–2mm
4. Confirm negative aspiration
5. Inject 3–5 mls of ropivacaine 0.5% or bupivacaine 0.25% at each level (4)

Note: Never advance the needle beyond 2.5cm due to risk of spinal cord injury.

Needle should be directed slightly posterior and caudad, never cephalad.

Paraesthesia is often elicited but is not specific enough to confirm the correct needle placement.

Total 20 marks

Further reading

N Ladak, J Thompson; General or local anaesthesia for carotid endarterectomy? *Continuing Education in Anaesthesia Critical Care & Pain*, Volume 12, Issue 2, April 2012, Pages 92–96.
NYOSORA Nerve Block App; Cervical plexus block https://www.nysora.com

Question 2

A 74-year-old woman presents to the emergency department with a 24-hour history of severe abdominal pain and signs of septic shock. She has a history of transient ischaemic attack. Her drug history is clopidogrel. Erect chest X-ray shows a pneumoperitoneum. The surgeons request anaesthetic
review pending urgent laparotomy.

A. **What modifiable organizational factors contribute to poor outcomes in patients requiring
   emergency laparotomy?** (2 marks)

   1. Delays in access to, or reporting of investigations
   2. Lack of access to senior clinicians
   3. Delay in time to surgery   (2)

B. **Briefly describe 5 recommended standards of care for a high-risk patient from the third NELA
   report** (5 marks)

   1. CT scan reported before surgery
   2. Risk of death documented before surgery
   3. Arrival in theatre within a timescale appropriate to urgency
   4. Preoperative review by consultants (surgeon and anaesthetist)
   5. Consultants present in operating theatre (surgeon and anaesthetist)
   6. Admission directly to critical care postoperatively when risk of death >10% (NELA-tool)
   7. Assessment by a specialist in care of the older person for patients ≥70 years   (5)

C. **List 4 commonly quoted risk calculators used for general surgery patients undergoing
   emergency laparotomy** (4 marks)

   1. NELA risk calculator—recommended
   2. Physiological and Operative Severity Score for the enumeration of Mortality and Morbidity
      (p-POSSUM)
   3. Surgical Outcome Risk Tool (SORT)
   4. American College of Surgeons National Surgical Quality Improvement Program
      (ACS NSQIP)
   5. Acute Physiology, Age, Chronic Health Evaluation II (APACHE II)
   6. American Society of Anaesthesiologists (ASA) class

   Note: Must have both NELA and POSSUM for 2 of the marks. The NELA risk prediction tool
   has been shown to be more accurate than the P-POSSUM calculator for patients undergoing
   emergency laparotomy in the UK.   (4)

D. On further assessment, the patient has a prominent history of side effects due to high dose systemic opioids. What measures, additional to simple analgesics, can be considered to facilitate an opioid sparing anaesthetic technique in this patient? (4 marks)

1. Transversus abdominus plane blocks
2. Rectus sheath blocks +/− catheter
3. Intravenous lidocaine infusion
4. IV Ketamine
5. IV Magnesium
6. Wound catheter local anaesthetic infusion

Note: No marks for central neuraxial analgesia as contraindicated by clopidogrel in this patient.

(4)

E. What intraoperative targets are recommended during management of an emergency laparotomy patient with signs of septic shock? (5 marks)

System	Goals
Cardiovascular (2 marks)	1. Aim MABP >65mmHg 2. Cardiac output monitoring (e.g. pulse contour analysis or oesophageal doppler) to guide goal directed fluid therapy (GDFT) 3. Vasopressor infusion (noradrenaline 1st line) for hypotension resistant to fluids
Respiratory (3 marks)	1. Lung protective ventilation 6–8ml/kg tidal volume 2. Inflation pressure limited to 30cmH$_2$0 3. Optimum PEEP 4. Recruitment manoeuvres as indicated

(5)

Total 20 marks

Further reading

N Eugene, M Cripps; Development and internal validation of a novel risk adjustment model for adult patients undergoing emergency laparotomy surgery: the National Emergency Laparotomy Audit risk model. *British Journal of Anaesthesia*, Volume 4, 2018, Pages 739–748.

C Ilyas, J Ones, S Fortey; Management of the patient presenting for emergency laparotomy, *BJA Education*, Volume, 19, Issue 4, 2019, Pages 113–118.

NELA Risk Calculator https://data.nela.org.uk/riskcalculator/

DI Saunders, D Murray, CJ Peden; Variations in mortality after emergency laparotomy: the first report of the UK Emergency Laparotomy Network, *British Journal of Anaesthesia*, Volume 109, 2012, Pages 368–375.

Question 3

A 79-year-old, life-long smoker attends for preoperative assessment prior to right pneumonectomy.

A. **List the absolute and relative indications for placement of a double lumen tube in anaesthesia and critical care** (5 marks)

Absolute

1. Isolation of the lung to prevent contamination (e.g. abscess)
2. Isolation of the lung to prevent leak of gases (e.g. bronchopleural fistula)
3. Pneumonectomy

Relative

1. Oesophagectomy (for surgical access)
2. All other thoracic surgery (except pneumonectomy)   (5)

B. **List methods of preoperative respiratory assessment you may use in an adult to assess their suitability for pneumonectomy? Give threshold values where required** (5 marks)

1. History of shortness of breath during activities of daily living, during talking, during walking on flat or stairs
2. Oxygen saturation at rest >90%
3. Spirometry FEV1 >1.5L (or >30% predicted) for pneumonectomy
4. Transfer factor (TLCO <30% is high risk)
5. Functional segment count such as quantitative isotope scan (shows proportion of perfused areas to be lost)
6. Shuttle walk testing. Distance >400 m is predictive of good postoperative function
7. Cardiopulmonary exercise testing (CPET) to measure oxygen uptake (VO_2 max). Aim for >15 ml/kg/min for good function postoperatively

Note: Must include FEV_1 and TLCO for marks   (5)

Note: arterial blood gases (ABGs) not recommended. Hypercapnoea is not itself a contraindication to surgery

C. **How would you manage hypoxaemia during one-lung anaesthesia?** (8 marks)

1. Increase the FiO_2 to 100%
2. Check the tube position by auscultation and fibreoptic scope
3. Check the tube patency with suction catheter
4. CPAP 5–10cmH$_2$O to the non-dependent lung
5. PEEP 5–10cmH$_2$O to the dependent lung
6. Intermittent re-inflation of the non-dependent lung
7. Insufflate low flow oxygen to the non-dependent lung
8. Clamp the pulmonary artery to the non-dependent lung to reduce shunt   (8)

D. **What is ventilation-perfusion coupling (V/Q)? What does it achieve?** (2 marks)

V/Q coupling matches the amount of gas reaching the alveoli to the blood flow in the corresponding pulmonary capillaries (1 mark). It reduces physiological dead space. (1 mark)   (2)

Total 20 marks

Further reading

British Thoracic Society; Society of Cardiothoracic Surgeons of Great Britain Ireland Working Party; BTS guidelines on the selection of patients with lung cancer for surgery, *Thorax*, Volume 56, Issue 2, February 2001, Pages 89–108.

AC Guyton, JE Hall. *Guyton and Hall Textbook of Medical Physiology* 9th Edition. Unit VII: Respiration. Chapters 37–42. Philadelphia, PA: W.B. Saunders Company, 1996, Pages 477–544.

NICE guidance on surgical treatment of lung cancer. Updated March 2019 https://www.nice.org.uk/guidance/ng122/chapter/Recommendations#treatment

Question 4

A. **List 4 risk factors for pre-eclampsia** (4 marks)

1. Primiparous or new partner
1. Pre-eclampsia in previous pregnancy
2. BMI >30
3. Family history of pre-eclampsia
4. Previous IUD
5. Previous placental abruption
6. Age over 40
7. Twins or triplets   (4)

Note: Pre-existing hypertension is not a risk factor.

B. **List criteria used in the diagnosis of mild pre-eclampsia** (3 marks)

1. New onset and persisting hypertension of BP >140/ >90
1. Occurring after the 20th week of gestation
2. Significant proteinuria   (3)

Note: Peripheral oedema is not included in diagnostic criteria.

C. List 3 drugs and their doses you would use to treat hypertension *in the order* you would use them (3 marks)

Antihypertensive choice	Drug	Initial dose and route	Maintenance
1st (1 mark)	Labetalol	200mg PO or 50mg IV. Repeat after 15 mins if required	Infuse at max 160mg/hr
2nd (1 mark)	Nifedipine MR	20mg PO (not SL) repeat after 30 mins if required	10 mg MR daily
3rd (1 mark)	Hydralazine	5mg IV over 15 mins	Infusion 5mg/hr titrate to BP
4th (no marks)	L bupivacaine	If epidural sited	–
5th (no marks)	Magnesium	Only if severe pre-eclampsia diagnosed	–

(3)

D. Give 2 further signs or symptoms that define pre-eclampsia as being severe (2 marks)

Systemic problems with mother or baby including:

1. Renal insufficiency (elevated creatinine)
2. Deranged liver function with rises transaminases or right upper quadrant (RUQ) pain
3. Haematological conditions. Low platelets or HELLP
4. Neurological conditions including headache, seizures
5. Pulmonary oedema
6. Foetal growth restriction

(2)

E. Give details of the magnesium administration regimen used in severe pre-eclampsia? (2 marks)

1. 1st bolus: 4g IV over 15–20 mins
2. IV infusion of 1g/hr for 24hr

(2)

Note: Therapeutic range of magnesium is 5–7mg/dL or 2–4mmol/L.

F. List 3 signs or symptoms of magnesium toxicity? (3 marks)

1. Respiratory weakness or shortness of breath (must exclude pulmonary oedema)
2. Limb weakness/absent tendon jerks
3. Palpitations/arrythmia/chest pain
4. Nausea/vomiting

Note: Only 1 from each category accepted

(3)

G. **How should magnesium toxicity be managed?** (3 marks)

1. Stop magnesium infusion
2. Give 10mls 10% calcium gluconate IV
3. Monitor electrocardiogram (ECG), NBP or intra-aortic balloon pump (IABP), tendon reflexes, check magnesium level (3)

Total 20 marks

Further reading

NICE guidance; Hypertension in pregnancy, diagnosis and management CG 107 https://www.nice.org.uk/guidance/ng133

NHS website; Conditions A to Z, Pre-eclampsia, last reviewed June 2018 https://www.nhs.uk/conditions/pre-eclampsia/causes/

The Eclampsia Trial Collaborative Group; Which anticonvulsant for women with eclampsia? Evidence from the Collaborative Eclampsia Trial, *The Lancet*, Volume 345, 1995, Pages 1455–1463.

Question 5

A 39-year-old man is scheduled for the excision of a medulloblastoma from his posterior cranial fossa. He is to be in the sitting position for his surgery.

A. **List 3 contraindications to the sitting position** (3 marks)

1. Ventriculoatrial shunt
2. Right to left heart shunt
3. Patent foramen ovale
4. Uncontrolled hypertension
5. Severe autonomic dysfunction (3)

B. **What are the complications associated with surgery in the sitting position?** (3 marks)

1. Cardiovascular instability
2. Venous pooling can lead to hypotension
3. Direct stimulation of medulla, pons, cranial nerve nuclei can lead to hypo/hypertension, brady/tachycardia, or arrhythmia
4. Venous air embolism
5. Pneumocephalus
6. Macroglossia
7. Quadriplegia (3)

C. List 2 ways in which the risk of venous air embolism can be minimized (2 marks)

1. Use Trendelenburg tilt
2. Leg elevation
3. Optimize fluid status   (2)

D. Complete this table with the clinical features of venous air embolism? (8 marks)

Cardiovascular (4 marks)	1. Hypotension 2. Shock 3. Tachyarrhythmia 4. Myocardial ischaemia 5. Right heart failure 6. Cardiac arrest (4)
Respiratory (3 marks)	1. Wheeze 2. Crepitations 3. Sudden drop in end-tidal CO_2 4. Hypoxia 5. Hypercarbia (3)
CNS (1 mark)	1. Cerebral hypoperfusion 2. Stroke (1)

                                                                                                            (8)

E. List 4 specific monitors that can be used to detect venous air embolism during anaesthesia (4 marks)

1. Transoesophageal echocardiogram—most sensitive
2. Precordial doppler—most sensitive non-invasive device
3. Pulmonary artery catheter to measure pulmonary artery and right atrial pressure
4. Oesophageal stethoscope—mill wheel murmur. Very insensitive test
5. End-tidal carbon dioxide—set tight limits so a sudden drop is detected
6. ECG changes such as arrhythmias, right heart strain, or ST depression can also help in the diagnosis   (4)

Total 20 marks

Further reading

S Jagannathan, H Krovvidi; Anaesthetic considerations for posterior fossa surgery, *Continuing Education in Anaesthesia Critical Care & Pain*, Volume 14, Issue 5, October 2014, Pages 202–206.

Question 6

A 49-year-old woman requires elective total thyroidectomy. She has a history of hyperthyroidism and Graves' disease. Her drug history includes carbimazole and propranolol.

A. **Give 2 clinical features which are specific to Graves' disease?** (2 marks)

1. Antithyroid-stimulating hormone (TSH) antibodies (positive in 80%)
2. Eye signs—exophthalmos
3. Pretibial myxoedema   (2)

B. **List 4 preoperative signs specific to goitre which may indicate potential airway difficulty during induction of anaesthesia** (4 marks)

1. Large neck swelling
2. Stridor
3. Tracheal deviation (clinically or CXR)
4. Unable to lie flat
5. Limited neck movement
6. Vena caval obstruction   (4)

C. **What clinical signs of hyperthyroidism can be detected at the bedside?** (4 marks)

System	Signs
CNS (1 marks)	1. Restlessness/anxiety 2. Tremor
CVS (2 marks)	1. Hypertension 2. Tachyarrhythmia 3. Atrial fibrillation 4. Cardiac failure signs
General (1 mark)	1. Weight loss/cachexia 2. Hyperhidrosis

(4)

D. **What are the biochemical indicators of hyperthyroid disease?** (1 mark)

Low TSH and high T3/T4 outside normal reference ranges

Note: Both required to receive the mark

(1)

E. During surgery the patient becomes acutely unwell. You suspect thyroid storm.

List 4 of the classical presenting features of thyroid storm (4 marks)

1. Usually occurs 6–24 hours post-surgery
2. Fever >40°C
3. Hyperhidrosis
4. Tachycardia >140bpm
5. Nausea/vomiting
6. Diarrhoea
7. Coma   (4)

F. Explain the importance of checking serum calcium postoperatively following total thyroid surgery? (1 mark)

To detect the rare complication of hypocalcaemia from unintentional removal of the parathyroid glands   (1)

G. Name the clinical signs which may be elicited on examination in this situation and describe their associated examination findings.

Clinical sign (2 marks)	**Examination findings** (2 marks)
1. Trousseau's sign	1. Carpopedal spasm precipitated by blood pressure cuff inflation
2. Chvostek's sign	2. Tapping over the facial nerve at the parotid causes facial twitching

(4)

Total 20 marks

Further reading

PA Farling; Thyroid disease, *BJA: British Journal of Anaesthesia*, Volume 85, Issue 1, 1 July 2000, Pages 15–28.
S Malhotra, V Sodhi; Anaesthesia for thyroid and parathyroid surgery, *Continuing Education in Anaesthesia Critical Care & Pain*, Volume 7, Issue 2, April 2007, Pages 55–58.

Question 7

A 6-year-old child presents with a dental abscess requiring surgery. She suffers from Down's syndrome. She has mild developmental delay and cannot cooperate with preoperative assessment.

A. Define Down's syndrome (2 marks)

1. Down's syndrome is a chromosomal disorder caused when an error in cell division results in an extra 21st chromosome, thus trisomy 21.
2. This leads to impaired cognitive ability, reduced physical growth, mild to moderate developmental disabilities, and a higher risk of some health problems (2)

Note: A syndrome is a collection of features hence the second part of definition is required.

B. List the airway issues relevant to the anaesthetic management of this particular child (6 marks)

Airway

1. Large tongue
2. Atlantoaxial instability
3. Inadequate pre-op assessment, mouth opening
4. Hypersalivation from protruding tongue
5. Shared airway (3)

General

1. Mouth opening may be limited by pain or trismus
2. Contaminated airway
3. Potential for difficult airway but difficult to quantify preoperatively
4. Fasting status unknown (3)

C. Give 2 options for induction of anaesthesia (1 mark)

1. IV induction/RSI
2. Gas induction (1)

D. Complete the table evaluating the risks and benefits of each method (8 marks)

Technique	Pros (4 marks)	Cons (4 marks)
IV induction/ RSI	1. Safe, quick, familiar, 2. Predictable 3. Optimizes intubation conditions (2)	1. Airway not evaluated 2. CICV situation may arise 3. Need IV access preinduction 4. Nasal intubation required for procedure 5. Preoxygenation may not be tolerated (2)

Technique	Pros (4 marks)	Cons (4 marks)
Gas induction	1. SV maintained 2. No IV access required 3. Child may be familiar with this technique. (2)	1. Slower 2. Mask may be painful on face or poor seal 3. Child may be uncooperative 4. Limited time for laryngoscopy and intubation 5. May not be fasted 6. Allows time for asleep fibreoptic intubation if required. (2)

(8)

E. Give 3 postoperative considerations (3 marks)

1. Airway obstruction: swelling or bleeding
2. Pain assessment and control
3. Needs monitored in HDU
4. May need to return to theatre
5. May require tracheostomy (3)

Total 20 marks

Further reading

L Abeysundara, A Creedon, D Soltanifar; Dental knowledge for anaesthetists, *BJA Education*, Volume 16, Issue 11, 1 November 2016, Pages 362–368.
JE Allt, CJ Howell; Down's syndrome, *BJA CEPD Reviews*, Volume 3, Issue 3, 1 June 2003, Pages 83–86.

Question 8

A 29-year-old woman is ventilated in ICU. She was admitted 48 hours ago with community acquired pneumonia. She has a history of anorexia nervosa and depression. She weighs 46kg.

A. What are the effects of malnutrition in the critical care patient? (3 marks)

1. Impaired immune function and increased risk of sepsis
2. Poor wound healing
3. Muscle wasting (including respiratory)
4. Impaired ventilatory drive
5. Low mood (3)

B. You commence enteral feeding via the nasogastric route. What are the risk factors for developing refeeding syndrome in critical care patients? (4 marks)

1. Low BMI (<16 alone or <18.5 with another risk factor present)
2. Unintentional weight loss >10–15% in the last 3–6 months
3. Little or no oral intake for more than 5–10 days
4. Critically low electrolyte levels on admission (potassium, phosphate, and magnesium)
5. History of alcohol or drugs including insulin, chemotherapy, and diuretics   (4)

C. Describe the metabolic changes that occur in refeeding syndrome (3 marks)

1. Feeding malnourished patients initiates a shift from the free fatty acid metabolism of starvation back to carbohydrate metabolism
2. Increased phosphate and thiamine requirements
3. Acute thiamine deficiency
4. Release of insulin
5. Intracellular shift of potassium, magnesium, and phosphate   (3)

D. List 6 clinical features of refeeding syndrome (6 marks)

1. Hypotension
2. Arrhythmias
3. Cardiac failure
4. Peripheral and pulmonary oedema
5. Lactic acidosis
6. Respiratory muscle weakness
7. Immune dysfunction
8. Seizures, coma
9. Neurological damage (e.g. Wernicke's encephalopathy or Korsakoff's psychosis)   (6)

E. What are the NICE recommendations for nutrition in patients at high risk of developing refeeding syndrome? (4 marks)

1. Start feeding at a maximum of 10kcal/kg/day increasing slowly to meet or exceed needs by day 4–7
2. Restore circulatory volume and monitor fluid status carefully
3. For the first 10 days of feeding give either full dose IV vitamin B preparation (Pabrinex) or oral thiamine 200–300mg daily with a balanced multivitamin and trace element supplement
4. Provide potassium, phosphate, and magnesium supplements daily, and monitor levels   (4)

Total 20 marks

Further reading

NICE guidance; Nutrition support for adults: oral nutrition support, enteral tube feeding and parenteral nutrition, Last updated Aug 2017 https://www.nice.org.uk/Guidance/CG32

P Singer, MM Berger, G Van den Berghe, et al. ESPEN guidelines on parenteral nutrition: intensive care. *Clinical Nutrition*, Volume 28, 2009, Pages 387–400.

Question 9

A 61-year-old unknown male is admitted to the intensive care unit because of deteriorating conscious level. He is intubated and ventilated. The neurology team have recommended further investigation with MRI of the head.

A. **What logistical challenges are faced by the anaesthetist taking an intensive care patient for MRI scan?** (5 marks)

1. Specific training/knowledge of MRI environment essential
2. Patient will require a transfer and remote site anaesthesia
3. Transfer onto non-standard monitoring and anaesthetic equipment
4. Long durations of MRI scan, sometimes up to 2 hours
5. Limited access to the patient due to cylindrical bore design
6. Technique should ensure the patient remains very still to avoid image artefact
7. In the event of emergency deterioration, patient will need to be removed from the scanning room

(5)

B. **What magnetic field strengths are typically used in an MRI scanner?** (1 mark)

0.5–3 Tesla (most operate at 1.5T)

Note: Must also state units to receive mark

(1)

C. **What is the fringe field** (1 mark) **and its significance?** (2 marks)

1. This is the peripheral magnetic field outside the magnetic core. It is delineated as a safety boundary. This smaller field is usually described in Gauss (G) (1)

1. The fringe field may cause interference in electronic devices
2. No patient or staff member should pass the 5G boundary without undergoing an MRI safety check
3. Anaesthesia should always be induced outside the 5G contour and adjacent to the scanner. This permits availability of standard equipment if required at induction of anaesthesia

Note: Ferromagnetic objects closer to the magnetic core, within a 30G (3mT) field, will experience an attractive force. Fields below 30G are generally insufficient to move unrestrained ferromagnetic objects. The boundary of 5G and below is considered 'safe' levels of static magnetic field exposure for the general public

(2)

D. The patient has now been transferred to the anaesthetic room outside the MRI scanner. Briefly describe 5 of the steps which should be performed to ensure the patient remains safe before entering the magnetic field (5 marks)

1. MRI safety checklist completed for the patient
2. Staff are safety checked and pockets empty
3. MR conditional anaesthetic machine checked and set up. Ensure monitoring is changed to MR conditional or remains outside room. Ensure all probes and cables are MR conditional including switching ECG dots to MR safe
4. All MR unsafe devices and equipment removed from patient, ensure syringe pumps are MR conditional
5. Patient transferred onto MR safe trolley or undocked scanner table
6. Tracheal tube pilot balloon is taped away from the head area to be scanned (ferromagnetic spring in the valve will cause artefact on images)
7. Hearing protection applied to the patient (5)

E. Outline the potential MRI-specific hazards to this patient inside the scanning room (5 marks)

1. Ferromagnetic objects may become dangerous projectiles attracted towards the centre of the magnetic field
2. Metal foreign bodies in tissue may become dislodged, leading to damage or haemorrhage; this is a particular hazard in the eye or close to blood vessels
3. Gradient fields—these induce a current in the body sufficient for stimulation of peripheral nerve and muscle cells
4. Acoustic noise—switching of fields causes loud noises, typically above the safe level for hearing of 80–85dB
5. Heating from radiofrequency fields—risk of burns from conductive material left on the patient's skin
6. Implanted pacemakers, defibrillators, neurostimulators, and other devices may be inactivated, reprogrammed, dislodged, or converted to an asynchronous mode by the magnetic field

Note: No marks for helium escape/quenching hypoxic environment as patient is ventilated artificially in a closed circuit

(5)

F. Describe the problem encountered following spontaneous or emergency shutdown of the magnetic field (1 mark)

Around 1,000L of liquid helium is used to keep the superconductor cool. In the event of an emergency shutdown of the magnetic field the helium expands to a gas (quenching) and must be vented out of the scan room quickly to prevent a hypoxic environment for all personnel (1)

Total 20 marks

Further reading

U Reddy, MJ White, SR Wilson; Anaesthesia for magnetic resonance imaging, *Continuing Education in Anaesthesia Critical Care & Pain*, Volume 12, Issue 3, 2012, Pages 140–144.

SR Wilson, S Shinde, I Appleby, et al.; Guidelines for the safe provision of anaesthesia in magnetic resonance units 2019, *Anaesthesia*, Volume 74, 2019, Pages 638–650.

Question 10

A 9-year-old child requires anaesthesia for appendicectomy. He has been vomiting and you plan a rapid sequence induction.

A. What is the physiological basis of preoxygenation for anaesthesia? (2 marks)

1. Replaces air (N_2/O_2) in the functional residual capacity (FRC) with oxygen
2. FRC then acts as O_2 store, increasing the time to hypoxaemia and desaturation allowing time for intubation/securing airway   (2)

B. What are the advantages and disadvantages of preoxygenating a child in this scenario? (4 marks)

Advantages (2 marks)	Disadvantages (2 marks)
1. Increases time to desaturation which is faster in a child 2. Reduces need for positive pressure ventilation before airway protected	1. Poorly tolerated by some children 2. Need a co-operative patient (difficult if the child is agitated) 3. Child is best placed on trolley, not on parents' knee 4. Seal can be difficult to achieve due to tears, saliva

(4)

C. How you would assess the efficacy of preoxygenation? (3 marks)

1. Ensure good facemask seal clinically
2. Ensure normal capnography trace
3. Aim for end-tidal O_2 concentration >85%
4. Aim for O_2 saturations 100%
5. Absence of desaturation during intubation   (3)

D. Label the 4 cartilaginous structures within the larynx indicated on the diagram (4 marks)

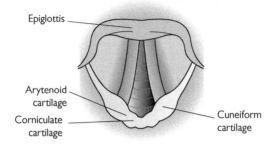

Epiglottis

Arytenoid
cartilage

Corniculate
cartilage

Cuneiform
cartilage

1. Epiglottis
2. Arytenoid cartilage
3. Corniculate cartilage
4. Cuneiform cartilage   (4)

E. Name the remaining 2 unpaired cartilages of the larynx (2 marks)

1. Thyroid cartilage
2. Cricoid cartilage   (2)

F. At the end of the operation you extubate the child. The abdomen is moving but no airflow is detected at the mouth. You diagnose laryngospasm.

Outline the pathophysiology of laryngospasm (5 marks)

1. Stimulus of the vocal cords during light anaesthesia causes laryngospasm
2. Afferent limb: sensory fibres travel via the internal branch of the superior laryngeal nerve to the vagus nerve
3. Efferent limb: the motor response is adduction of the vocal cords via 3 intrinsic muscles of the larynx—the lateral cricoarytenoids, the thyroarytenoids (glottic adductors), and cricoarytenoids (glottic tensors)
4. These muscles are supplied by the vagus nerve via the recurrent laryngeal nerve
5. Response is adduction of the cords   (5)

Total 20 marks

Further reading

G Gavel, RWM Walker; Laryngospasm in anaesthesia, *Continuing Education in Anaesthesia Critical Care & Pain*, Volume 14, Issue 2, April 2014, Pages 47–51.

Question 11

You are asked to urgently assess a 2-year-old boy in the emergency department who has stridor of acute onset over 2–3 hours. He is sitting upright with suprasternal and subcostal recession. He has no medical history.

A. **What is the definition of stridor?** (2 marks)

1. Stridor is an abnormal noise heard on inspiration
2. It is caused by turbulent air flow through a narrowed airway (2)

B. **Why are paediatric airways more prone to stridor than in adults?** (2 marks)

1. Paediatric airways are smaller—a small decrease in the radius of the airway results in a marked increase in resistance to airflow and the work of breathing (Poiseuille's law)
2. More prone to occlusion by secretions or oedema
3. Cartilaginous support components are less developed and more compliant (e.g. tracheal tug) (2)

C. **List discriminating features of the differential diagnoses provided** (13 marks)

Croup (3 marks)	1. Most common (approx. 80% of cases) 2. Classic barking cough (often described as like a seal) 3. Low grade fever 4. Improved by adrenaline nebulizer
Epiglottitis (3 marks)	1. Sore throat/drooling/dysphagia 2. Very unwell child with high fever 3. Absence of cough 4. Usually not improved by adrenaline nebulizer
Anaphylaxis (2 marks)	1. History of allergy 2. History of exposure to a known trigger 3. Other coexisting systemic features of anaphylaxis
Inhaled foreign body (2 marks)	1. Sudden onset, no prodromal illness 2. High index of suspicion or timing suggestive (e.g. onset eating food at mealtime)
Bacterial tracheitis (3 marks)	1. Rare 2. Constitutionally unwell, high fever 3. Coughing with copious tracheal secretions 4. No dysphagia or drooling 5. Able to lie flat

(13)

D. Briefly describe 3 main principles in the management of croup (3 marks)

1. Medical management—steroids and nebulized adrenaline
2. Avoid distressing the child which could worsen airway obstruction
3. Airway management/planning (e.g. senior clinicians, ENT surgeon immediately available)
4. Intubation in theatre environment if possible (3)

Total 20 marks

Further reading

E Maloney, GH Meakin; Acute stridor in children, *Continuing Education in Anaesthesia Critical Care & Pain*, Volume 7, Issue 6, 2007, Pages 183–186.

Question 12

A 76-year-old lady presents with an infected hip replacement. She is scheduled for a revision hip replacement. You intend to use cell salvage as part of your perioperative management.

A. Describe the process of cell salvage from surgical site to reinfusion of red cells to the patient (5 marks)

1. Collect blood from the operative site via low pressure suction catheter
2. Mixed with anticoagulant as it is aspirated into a collection reservoir
3. Passed through a filter
4. Once enough blood has been collected (>500ml usually) processing begins
5. Red cells are separated from whole anticoagulated blood by centrifugation
6. Red cells are washed with sterile saline 0.9% and the effluent siphoned off to waste
7. Processed red cells suspended in saline 0.9% at a high haematocrit are pumped to a sterile reinfusion bag (5)

B. What specific considerations are there for cell salvage in this particular patient? (3 marks)

1. NICE guidelines recommend that cell salvage should not be used routinely without also administering tranexamic acid
2. Cell salvage suctioning must not occur when cement is being applied but can be resumed once this is concluded
3. Cell salvage should not be contaminated with topical antibiotics, iodine, or clotting agents but can be resumed when they are washed away
4. For revision surgery there is evidence the 40micron filters do not eliminate the smallest fragments of titanium so caution is advised for use with revision procedures (3)

C. You also intend to use TEG as part of your management.

What is TEG? (2 marks)

It is a point-of-care (bedside) analysis (1 mark) and display of the visco-elastic properties of a whole blood sample, from fibrin formation to clot retraction and fibrinolysis (1 mark)   (2)

D. What are the limitations of TEG? (4 marks)

1. Poor at detecting conditions affecting platelet adhesion
2. Preoperative baseline TEG is a poor predictor of postoperative bleeding
3. Will not reflect the effects of hypothermia on coagulation
4. Insensitive to the effects of clopidogrel and aspirin
5. May not be adequately maintained and requires quality control, training, and supervision outwith the laboratory environment
6. More expensive than laboratory testing   (4)

E. Identify and describe the clinical significance of the following parameters obtained from a TEG in the following table (6 marks)

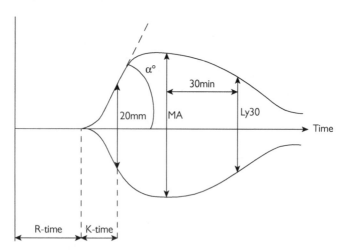

Reproduced from *SAQs for the Final FRCA*, Shorthouse J et al., Figure 3. Copyright Oxford University Press, 2011. Reproduced with permission of the Licensor through PLSclear.

	Name	Description
R (2 marks)	Reaction-Time (1)	Indicates concentration of soluble clotting factors in the plasma. Correlates with activated partial thromboplastin time (APTT) and PT (1)
α angle (2 marks)	Alpha angle (1)	Represents acceleration of fibrin build up and crosslinking (1)
MA (2 marks)	Maximum amplitude (1)	Represents ultimate strength of clot and depends on the number and function of platelets and the fibrinogen concentration (1)

(6)

Total 20 marks

Further reading

Association of Anaesthetists of Great Britain and Ireland Guidelines; Cell salvage for peri-operative blood conservation 2018 https://anaesthetists.org/Home/Resources-publications/Guidelines/Cell-salvage-for-peri-operative-blood-conservation-2018

A Srivastava, A Kelleher; Point-of-care coagulation testing, *Continuing Education in Anaesthesia Critical Care & Pain*, Volume 13, Issue 1, February 2013, Pages 12–16.

Exam 6 **Questions**

Exam 6 contains 12 selected Constructed Response Questions (CRQs) balanced across the intermediate curriculum, reflecting the Final Examination of the Diploma of Fellowship of the Royal
College of Anaesthetists (FRCA) exam. We recommend attempting these questions under exam
conditions. Please limit/contain your answer to/within the dotted lines given for each question.

Question 1

A. Complete the table describing pain changes between the first and second stages of labour
   (6 marks)

	1st stage	2nd stage
Source of pain	Uterine contraction and cervical dilation (3 marks)	Head in birth canal (3 marks)
Type of pain		
Afferent nerve type/speed		
Spinal dermatome level		

B. Describe the central pain pathway associated with the perception of labour pain. Begin at
   entry to the spinal cord (5 marks)

C. Name 3 areas of the brain involved in perception of pain (3 marks)

1. ....

2. ....

3. ....

D. Give 2 examples of important variables determining the perception of pain (2 marks)

1. ....

2. ....

E. Why is a higher dermatomal level of regional block required for Caesarean section than for analgesia in labour? (1 mark)

....

....

F. List the causes of bradycardia during regional anaesthesia for caesarean section (3 marks)

1. ....

2. ....

3. ....

Total 20 marks

Question 2

A 32-year-old woman with acute intermittent porphyria (AIP) presents for an open reduction and internal fixation (ORIF) of fractured right tibia and fibula.

A. What is the pathogenesis of AIP? (3 marks)

....

....

....

....

B. List the specific preoperative assessment and management of this patient (7 marks)

....

....

....

....

....

....

....

....

C. List 4 commonly used anaesthetic drugs that should be avoided in patients with AIP as they are potentially porphyrogenic (4 marks)

1. ....

2. ....

3. ....

4. ....

D. Surgery proceeds uneventfully under general anaesthesia. However, 30 minutes after arrival in recovery you are called back to see the patient. She has a heart rate of 134bpm, blood pressure is 179/94mmHg. She is complaining of severe abdominal pain and nausea.

You suspect an acute porphyric crisis and call for help.

Outline your initial (4 marks) and secondary (2 marks) management.

....

....

....

....

....

....

....

....

....

Total 20 marks

Question 3

You are asked to review a 71-year-old man in preoperative assessment. He is listed for laparoscopic assisted right hemicolectomy for bowel adenocarcinoma. His haemoglobin is 98g/dL. He is suitable for enhanced recovery after colorectal surgery protocols.

A. **What is the definition of anaemia? Include the differences between male and female sex**
(2 marks)

....

....

B. **You suspect absolute iron deficiency anaemia in this patient. List 6 likely findings on full blood count and haematinics** (6 marks)

1. ....

2. ....

3. ....

4. ....

5. ....

6. ....

C. What options for preoperative optimization are available for his anaemia? (4 marks)

1. ....

2. ....

3. ....

4. ....

D. What are the indications for preoperative intravenous iron therapy in anaemia? (2 marks)

1. ....

2. ....

E. What intraoperative techniques can be employed to minimize blood loss during this surgery? (2 marks)

1. ....

2. ....

F. How is acute pain usually managed for laparoscopic colorectal surgery as part of an enhanced recovery regime? (4 marks)

1. ....

2. ....

3. ....

4. ....

Total 20 marks

Question 4

A previously well 25-year-old man is brought to the emergency department (ED) at 03.00hrs. He has had a witnessed seizure in a nightclub and an ambulance was called. His Glasgow Coma Scale (GCS) is 6 on arrival and he is sweating.

A. What is your differential diagnosis? (5 marks)

1. ....

2. ....

3. ....

4. ....

5. ....

B. What is your initial management of this patient? (4 marks)

1. ....

2. ....

3. ....

4. ....

C. A bottle of dosulepin is found in his pocket. You suspect an overdose. His tympanic temperature is 38.1°C and you diagnose serotonin syndrome.

What classes of drugs can increase serotonin levels? Give examples of each (3 marks)

1. ....

2. ....

3. ....

D. Complete the table to show the symptoms of serotonin syndrome prior to seizure and coma (6 marks)

CNS (3 marks)	1. ....
	2. ....
	3. ....
CVS (1 mark)	1. ....
GI (2 marks)	1. ....
	2. ....

E. Regarding neuroleptic malignant syndrome, state the class of drugs most often implicated and the pathophysiology of the syndrome (2 marks)

....

....

Total 20 marks

Question 5

A 78-year-old man presents with a ruptured abdominal aortic aneurysm, confirmed on computed tomography (CT) scan. You are called to see him in the ED of a hospital with vascular surgery on-site. His GCS is 15 and he has a heart rate of 110bpm and a blood pressure of 87/45mmHg.

A. Outline your immediate preoperative assessment and management in the ED (7 marks)

....

....

....

....

....

....

....

....

B. The patient proceeds to theatre and is anaesthetised uneventfully. He loses 2 litres of blood during the first hour of surgery. You activate the major haemorrhage protocol and he requires transfusion of 8 units packed red cells and 4 pools of fresh frozen plasma.

What are the complications of massive blood transfusion? (5 marks)

1. ....

2. ....

3. ....

4. ....

5. ....

C. The surgeon gains control of bleeding and surgery proceeds. An hour later the surgeon says they are about the un-clamp the aorta.

Outline the haemodynamic and metabolic changes that lead to hypotension with aortic cross-clamp release (5 marks)

....

....

....

....

....

D. How can you attenuate this response? (3 marks)

....

....

....

Total 20 marks

Question 6

A 55-year-old builder attends the pain clinic with a 10-year history of back pain. It travels down the back of his thigh on the left side.

A. What is the diagnosis? (1 mark)

1. ....

B. Name 5 aspects of his chronic back pain that are important to elicit? (5 marks)

1. ....

2. ....

3. ....

4. ....

5. ....

C. How would you assess the impact the pain is having on his life? (4 marks)

1. ....

2. ....

3. ....

4. ....

D. What other aspects of his life may affect his pain? (3 marks)

....

....

....

....

E. What pharmacological therapies would you recommend? (2 marks)

....

....

....

F. Give 5 non-pharmacological therapies that may be useful? (5 marks)

1. ....

2. ....

3. ....

4. ....

5. ....

Total 20 marks

Question 7

A 42-year-old man presents for a nephrectomy. He is known to have dilated cardiomyopathy (DCM).

A. Describe the pathophysiology of evolving DCM? (2 marks)

....

....

....

B. What are the clinical features of DCM? (4 marks)

1. ....

2. ....

3. ....

4. ....

C. List 2 of the commonest causes of DCM in the UK (2 marks)

1. ....

2. ....

D. List 3 classes of drug, each with an example, that are used in the medical management of DCM (6 marks)

Drug class (3 marks)	**Example** (3 marks)

E. List 2 non-pharmacological options to manage advanced heart failure secondary to DCM? (2 marks)

1. ....

2. ....

F. The patient presents for his surgery. List the cardiovascular goals when anaesthetising this patient (4 marks)

1. ....

2. ....

3. ....

4. ....

Total 20 marks

Question 8

A 39-year-old man is unconscious in the ED. He was pulled from a house fire by the emergency services. He has a past medical history of schizophrenia and alcohol excess. On examination the man has burns to his torso and legs amounting to 30% total body surface area. He weighs 80kg. There is no evidence of significant trauma on the primary survey.

A. State the Parkland formula, calculate his resuscitation fluid requirements for the initial 24 hours and state how quickly this is administered (4 marks)

....

....

....

....

B. What aspects of the history from the paramedics would be associated with an increased risk of smoke inhalation injury? (2 marks)

....

....

C. What are the signs and symptoms of smoke inhalation injury? (6 marks)

1. ....

2. ....

3. ....

4. ....

5. ....

6. ....

D. The patient remains GCS 5. He has no obvious facial burns or swelling. His PaO_2 is 11kPa on 15L oxygen via a trauma mask and his carboxyhaemoglobin level is 20%. You plan to intubate the patient.

What differences and potential challenges must you be aware of when compared with a standard rapid sequence induction? (6 marks)

....

....

....

....

....

....

....

....

E. What 2 findings on his arterial blood gases and U&Es would suggest significant cyanide poisoning? (2 marks)

1. ....

2. ....

Total 20 marks

Question 9

You anaesthetise a 29-year-old man for an urgent appendicectomy. He is ASA1 and has had a previous anaesthetic for an ORIF right wrist with no problems. You perform a rapid sequence induction uneventfully with propofol and suxamethonium. Five minutes after knife to skin you note his etCO$_2$ has increased to 9kPA and his heart rate is 121bpm. You suspect malignant hyperthermia (MH).

A. List 5 other potential differential diagnoses (5 marks)

1. ....

2. ....

3. ....

4. ....

5. ....

B. On re-assessment his blood pressure is 81/45mmHg, his heart rate is 130bpm, his core temperature is 39.8°C, and his etCO$_2$ is now 9.8kPa.

List 5 additional clinical signs that would indicate a classical MH presentation (5 marks)

1. ....

2. ....

3. ....

4. ....

5. ....

C. You declare a critical incident, halt surgery, and call for help.

Outline your acute management to halt the MH process (6 marks)

....

....

....

....

....

....

....

D. Outline the aetiology of MH (3 marks)

....

....

....

....

E. What is the mechanism of action of dantrolene? (1 mark)

....

....

Total 20 marks

Question 10

A 6-year-old 20kg boy has sustained an open eye injury with associated threat of sight loss. He requires urgent examination under anaesthesia.

A. Describe the mechanism of further sight loss following the primary open eye injury, preoperatively? (2 marks)

....

....

....

B. Complete the table regarding the influence of anaesthetic factors on intraocular pressure
(5 marks)

Factor	Influence on IOP	Mechanism
15° head up tilt (1 mark)		
IV induction agent (1 mark)		
Depolarising muscle relaxant (1 mark)		
Laryngoscopy (1 mark)		
Hypocapnia (pCO$_2$ 3.5–4.0 kPa) (1 mark)		

C. Following commencement of the procedure in theatre, the patient develops severe bradycardia. Describe the oculo-cardiac reflex arc by completing the table (7 marks).

Trigger (1 mark)	
Afferent arc (2 marks)	
Efferent arc (2 marks)	
Effects (2 marks)	

D. The surgeon begins to examine the child under anaesthetic. The heart rate drops to 21 beats per minute. Outline in detail the immediate management (3 marks).

1. ....

2. ....

3. ....

E. Briefly describe 3 ways to further reduce the likelihood of adverse oculo-medullary reflexes in this case? (3 marks)

1. ....

2. ....

3. ....

Total 20 marks

Question 11

A 74-year-old man presents for an elective triple vessel coronary artery bypass (CABG).

A. List 6 patient related factors that are used in the European System for Cardiac Operative Risk Evaluation (EUROScore2) (6 marks)

1. ....

2. ....

3. ....

4. ....

5. ....

6. ....

B. The surgeon is performing the operation on cardiopulmonary bypass.

List the components of a basic cardiopulmonary bypass circuit (6 marks)

C. List 2 functions of cardioplegia in cardiac surgery? (2 marks)

1.

2.

D. The surgery proceeds uneventfully using cardiopulmonary bypass and hypothermia.

Outline your preparation in anticipation of weaning this patient from cardiopulmonary bypass (6 marks)

Total 20 marks

Question 12

A 54-year-old male patient is listed as an emergency to receive cadaveric renal transplantation. He has end stage renal failure, maintained on haemodialysis.

A. List 4 of the most common primary causes of end stage renal failure in the UK? (4 marks)

1. ....

2. ....

3. ....

4. ....

B. How is chronic kidney disease (CKD) classified? (2 marks)

1. ....

2. ....

C. What factors inform the assessment of this patient's dialysis dependency preoperatively? (5 marks)

1. ....

2. ....

3. ....

4. ....

5. ....

D. What are the indications for dialysis before transplantation? (3 marks)

1. ....

2. ....

3. ....

E. What potential problems are presented by recent dialysis if proceeding to surgery immediately after its completion? (2 marks)

1. ....

2. ....

F. The patient has a functional arteriovenous fistula (AVF) in his right forearm.

How should the AVF sites be protected intraoperatively? (4 marks)

1. ....

2. ....

3. ....

4. ....

Total 20 marks

Exam 6 **Answers**

Many of the following questions contain more answers than there are marks allocated. This redundancy is intentional and is to ensure that a spread of possible answers by the candidate are recognized. 1 mark is awarded per correct point up to the maximum specified in each subsection.

Question 1

A. Complete the table describing the pain changes between the first and second stages of labour (6 marks)

	1st stage	**2nd stage**
Source of pain	Uterine contraction and cervical dilation (3 marks)	Head in birth canal (3 marks)
Type of pain	Diffuse/visceral/dull	Localized/somatic/sharp
Afferent nerve type/speed	Small slow unmyelinated C fibres via sympathetic afferents	Fast fine myelinated A delta fibres (via pudendal nerve)
Spinal dermatome level	T10–L2	S2–S4

(6)

B. Describe the pain pathway associated with the perception of labour pain. Begin at entry to the spinal cord (5 marks)

1. Primary afferents pass via the sympathetic chain
2. Enter spinal cord at T10–L1
3. Synapse in the dorsal horn
4. Decussate and ascend to the brain via the spinothalamic tract
5. Reach the thalamus and the higher brain centres
(5)

C. Name 3 other areas of the brain involved in the perception of pain (3 marks)

1. Thalamus (only if not given in part B)
1. Primary and secondary somatosensory cortex
1. Amygdala
2. Prefrontal cortex
3. Insula
4. Anterior cingulate gyrus
5. Hippocampus

Note: No marks for areas mentioned in part 2 or for stating 'higher centres' or 'pain matrix'
(3)

D. Give 2 examples of important variables in determining the perception of pain (2 marks)

1. Memory
2. Past experience
3. Mood
4. Cognition
5. Beliefs
6. Gender
7. Emotions (2)

E. Why is a higher dermatomal level of regional block required for caesarean section than for analgesia in labour? (1 mark)

Caesarean section requires block of the peritoneum which takes a relatively high innervation from levels up to T4 having descended during embryological development (1)

F. List the causes of bradycardia during regional anaesthesia for caesarean section (3 marks)

1. Bradycardia occurring secondary to the unopposed parasympathetic stimulation of peritoneal stretch
2. Block of sympathetic cardio-accelerator fibres during a high block from T1 to T4 level sympathetic nerves
3. Use of phenylephrine infusion as a vasopressor causing a reflex bradycardia
4. Vaso-vagal episode/anxiety
5. Rapid onset of spinal block

(3)

Total 20 marks

Further reading

S Labor, S Maguire; The pain of labour, *Reviews in Pain*, Volume 2, Issue 2, December 2008, Pages 15–19.
M Serpell; Anatomy, physiology and pharmacology of pain, *Surgery*, Volume 24, Issue 10, 2006, Pages 350–353.

Question 2

A 32 year old woman with AIP presents for an ORIF of fractured right tibia and fibula.

A. What is the pathogenesis of AIP? (3 marks)

1. It is an inherited disorder of the haem biosynthesis pathway
2. It demonstrates autosomal dominant inheritance with variable expression
3. The genetic defect causes a deficiency of the enzyme porphobilinogen **(PBG) deaminase** (3)

B. List the specific preoperative assessment and management of this patient (7 marks)

1. Full medical history including family history
2. Details of previous acute crises and precipitating causes
3. Full examination including neurological
4. Assess for symptoms or signs of peripheral neuropathy or autonomic instability
5. Document any neurological deficit carefully especially if planning a regional technique
6. Senior anaesthetic involvement
7. Multidisciplinary team (MDT) approach with medical team and pharmacy
8. Ensure minimal fasting period
9. Consider intravenous dextrose10%/saline to avoid calorie restriction
10. Consider anxiolytic premedication (anxiety and stress can provoke an acute crisis)   (7)

C. List 4 commonly used anaesthetic drugs that should be avoided in patients with AIP as they are potentially porphyrogenic (4 marks)

1. Ketamine
2. Thiopentone
3. Sevoflurane
4. Ephedrine
5. Oxycodone
6. Diclofenac
7. Metaraminol (effects of metaraminol are undetermined so caution with its use is advised)   (4)

D. Surgery proceeds uneventfully under general anaesthesia. However, 30 minutes after arrival in recovery you are called back to see the patient. She has a heart rate of 134bpm, blood pressure is 179/94mmHg. She is complaining of severe abdominal pain and nausea.

You suspect an acute porphyric crisis and call for help.

Outline your initial (4 marks) and secondary (2 marks) management.

Initial

1. Remove and treat any potential triggering factors
2. Give intravenous haem arginate as soon as possible. Continue for 4 days
3. Titrate morphine to pain. Paracetamol is also safe
4. Consider patient controlled analgesia for ongoing pain control. Often there are very high requirements so standard settings may not be enough
5. Antiemetic: ondansetron and prochlorperazine are safe to use
6. Control tachycardia and hypertension with B-blockers if no contra-indications

Note: must have specific treatment with haem arginate for full marks   (4)

Secondary

1. Give iv dextrose 10%/saline 0.9% and consider oral or nasogastric carbohydrate loading to prevent catabolic state
2. Monitor U&Es and treat any hyponatraemia
3. Admit to high dependency unit (HDU) for ongoing supportive treatment and monitoring
4. Send urine for PBG (porphobilinogen) assay to confirm the diagnosis (2)

Total 20 marks

Further reading

The Drug Database for Acute Porphyria http://www.drugs-porphyria.org/
H Findley, A Philips, D Cole, A Nair; Porphyrias: implications for anaesthesia, critical care, and pain medicine, *Continuing Education in Anaesthesia Critical Care & Pain*, Volume 12, Issue 3, June 2012, Pages 128–133.

Question 3

You are asked to review a 71-year-old man in preoperative assessment. He is listed for laparoscopic assisted right hemicolectomy for bowel adenocarcinoma. His haemoglobin is 98g/L. He is suitable for enhanced recovery after colorectal surgery protocols.

A. What is the definition of anaemia? Include the differences between male and female sex (2 marks)

Anaemia is defined by the World Health Organization as a haemoglobin concentration <130g/L for men (1 mark), <120g/L non-pregnant women (1 mark) (and <110g/L for pregnant women) (2)

B. You suspect absolute iron deficiency anaemia in this patient. List 6 likely findings on full blood count and haematinics (6 marks)

1. Mean cell volume (MCV) low <80fL
2. Mean cell haemoglobin (MCH) low <27pg
3. Haematocrit low
4. Ferritin low <30mcg/L
5. Serum iron low
6. Transferrin saturation (TSAT) low <20%
7. High transferrin or total iron binding capacity (TIBC)
8. High platelet count
9. Low reticulocytes (6)

C. **What options for preoperative optimization are available for his anaemia?** (4 marks)

1. Dietary advice
2. Oral iron supplements
3. Additional vitamin C—improves iron absorption from the diet
4. Intravenous iron infusion
5. Preoperative red cell transfusion
6. Rule out/treat other coexisting causes of blood loss (4)

D. **What are the indications for preoperative intravenous iron therapy in anaemia?** (2 marks)

1. Failure to respond to, or to tolerate oral iron
2. Surgery to be expedited (e.g. cancer surgery) (2)

E. **What intraoperative techniques can be employed to minimize blood loss during this surgery?** (2 marks)

1. Surgical technique—meticulous attention to blood loss
2. Completion laparoscopically, avoiding an open procedure (2)

F. **How is acute pain usually managed for laparoscopic colorectal surgery as part of an enhanced recovery regime?** (4 marks)

1. Single shot spinal anaesthesia preferred
2. Intrathecal opioid administered
3. Adjuncts considered: IV lidocaine, gabapentinoids, ketamine, and alpha$_2$-agonists all described
4. Regular paracetamol
5. Rescue analgesia (e.g. oxycodone PCA) (4)

Total 20 marks

Further reading

LJS Kelliher, CN Jones, WJ Fawcett; Enhanced recovery for gastrointestinal surgery. *Continuing Education in Anaesthesia Critical Care & Pain*, Volume 15, Issue 6, 2015, Pages 305—310.

M Munoz, AG Acheson, M Auerbach; International consensus statement on the peri-operative management of anaemia and iron deficiency. *Anaesthesia*, Volume 72, 2017, Pages 233–247.

SV Thakrar, B Clevenger, S Mallett; Patient blood management and perioperative anaemia, *BJA Education*, Volume 17, Issue 1, January 2017, Pages 28–34.

Question 4

A previously well 25-year-old man is brought to the ED at 03.00hrs. He has had a witnessed seizure in a nightclub and an ambulance was called. His GCS is 6 on arrival and he is sweating.

A. **What is your differential diagnosis?** (5 marks)

1. Epileptic seizure or first presentation of epilepsy
2. Head injury
3. Hypoglycaemia
4. Alcohol intoxication
5. Subarachnoid haemorrhage (SAH)
6. Drug overdose or reaction, prescribed or illegal
7. Neuroleptic malignant syndrome
8. Serotonin syndrome

Note: no mark given for serotonin syndrome, see part C. (5)

B. **What is your initial management of this patient?** (4 marks)

1. RSI, intubation
2. Ventilation to normalize physiology (pH and pCO_2)
3. Standard IV access and cooled IV fluids
4. Check blood glucose, pupils, arrange CT head, check temperature
5. Ensure safe environment in case of further seizures
6. *Consider* dantrolene, IV benzodiazepine, active cooling (4)

Note: For information only. No additional marks for these notes.
Treatment is supportive and the causative agent removed. Dantrolene has been used and may have some effect in reducing muscle rigidity but the evidence is case report only and its efficacy is not reliable. Haemofiltration may be considered at a later stage.

C. **A bottle of dosulepin is found in his pocket. His tympanic temperature is 38.1°C. An overdose is suspected and you diagnose serotonin syndrome.**

What classes of drugs can increase serotonin levels? Give examples of each (3 marks)

1. Antidepressants: SSRIs, SNRI, TCA (dosulepin), trazodone, and mirtazapine, St John's Wort
2. Analgesics: tramadol, fentanyl
3. Antiemetics: ondansetron and metoclopramide
4. Triptans (migraine): sumatriptan
5. Illegal drugs: ecstasy (MDMA), cocaine, and amphetamines
6. Methylene blue

Note: 1 from each of 3 different categories required for marks (3)

D. Complete the table to show the symptoms of serotonin syndrome prior to seizure and coma (6 marks)

CNS (3 marks)	1. Clonus (including ocular clonus) 2. Hyper-reflexia 3. Disorientation, confusion, anxiety 4. Hypertonicity 5. Pupil dilatation 6. Hallucinations (3)
CVS (1 mark)	1. Tachycardia 2. Hypertension (1)
GI (2 marks)	1. Nausea 2. Diarrhoea (2)

(6)

E. Regarding neuroleptic malignant syndrome, state the class of drugs most often implicated and the pathophysiology of the syndrome (2 marks)

1. Class of drugs: antipsychotics
2. Pathophysiology: antagonism of dopamine (DA2) receptors in the central nervous system (CNS) with side effects of drugs manifest via extrapyramidal pathways.

(2)

Total 20 marks

Further reading

S Chinniah, JL French, DM Levy; Serotonin and anaesthesia, *CEACCP*, Volume 8, Issue 2, 1 April 2008, Pages 43–45.
T Peck, A Wong, E Norman; Anaesthetic implications of psychoactive drugs, *Continuing Education in Anaesthesia Critical Care and Pain*, Volume 10, Issue 6, 1 December 2010, Pages 177–181.

Note: For information only. (No additional marks)

Serotonin syndrome is due to increased levels of serotonin in the synapse. It is also known as serotonin toxicity. It is diagnosed using Hunter's criteria (hyper-reflexia, clonus). In contrast, neuroleptic malignant syndrome is an idiosyncratic reaction to antipsychotic medication characterized by hyperthermia, autonomic dysfunction, and muscle rigidity. It has a 20–30% mortality. Treatment is supportive with dantrolene and non-depolarizing muscle relaxants (NDMR) being used to reduce muscle rigidity. It is more common with typical, rather than atypical antipsychotics.

Question 5

A 78-year-old man presents with a ruptured abdominal aortic aneurysm, confirmed on CT scan. You are called to see him in the ED of a hospital with vascular surgery on-site. His GCS is 15 and he has a heart rate of 110 bpm and a blood pressure of 87/45mmHg.

A. Outline your immediate preoperative assessment and management in the ED (7 marks)

1. Emergency situation so rapid evaluation imperative
2. Consideration to appropriateness of surgery, risk scoring (e.g. V-possum)
3. Call for Consultant vascular surgeon and Consultant anaesthetist
4. Brief targeted history and airway/anaesthetic assessment
5. 2 × wide bore cannula. Don't delay for invasive monitoring
6. Baseline FBC, COAG, and U&Es
7. Alert blood bank by activating the major haemorrhage protocol
8. Request crossmatched blood 8 units
9. Judicious fluid resuscitation to MAP ≤ 70mmHg
10. Alert theatre and ICU
11. Set up rapid infuser and cell salvage   (7)

B. The patient proceeds to theatre and is anaesthetised uneventfully. He loses 2L of blood during the first hour of surgery. You activate the major haemorrhage protocol and he requires transfusion of 8 units packed red cells and 4 pools of fresh frozen plasma. What are the complications of massive blood transfusion? (5 marks)

1. Dilutional coagulopathy
2. Hypothermia
3. Hyperkalaemia
4. Hypocalcaemia
5. Acidosis
6. Citrate toxicity
7. Transfusion-associated circulatory overload (TACO)
8. Transfusion-related acute lung injury (TRALI)   (5)

C. The surgeon gains control of bleeding and surgery proceeds. An hour later the surgeon says they are ready to un-clamp the aorta. Outline the haemodynamic and metabolic changes that lead to hypotension with aortic cross-clamp release (5 marks)

1. Sudden decrease in afterload due to a reduction in peripheral vascular resistance and vasodilatation when clamp released
2. Blood sequestration in lower half of body
3. Lactic acidosis
4. Ischaemic-reperfusion injury
5. Decreased myocardial contractility
6. Decreased cardiac output   (5)

D. **How can you attenuate this response?** (3 marks)

1. Expand circulating volume/volume loading prior to clamp release
2. Vasoconstrictors
3. Positive inotropic drugs
4. Increase FiO_2
5. Instruct surgeons to release the clamp gradually and re-clamp if necessary   (3)

Total 20 marks

Further reading

M Al-Hashimi, J Thompson; Anaesthesia for elective open abdominal aortic aneurysm repair, *Continuing Education in Anaesthesia Critical Care & Pain*, Volume 13, Issue 6, December 2013, Pages 208–212.

HP Phan, BH Shaz; Update on massive transfusion. *British Journal of Anaesthesia*, Volume 111, Supplement 1, December 2013, Pages i71–i82.

Question 6

A 55-year-old builder attends the pain clinic with a 10-year history of back pain. It travels down the back of his thigh on the left side.

A. **What is the diagnosis?** (1mark)

Biomechanical back pain.   (1)

Note: The diagnosis is not sciatica. Sciatic pain is defined as pain spreading below the knee, usually to the heel and foot.

B. **Name 5 aspects of his chronic back pain that are important to elicit?** (5 marks)

1. Red flags; urinary or bowel incontinence, weakness, a sudden increase in pain
2. Nature of pain (sharp, dull, burning, lancing, gnawing)
3. When and how it started
4. Aggravating and relieving factors
5. Associated sensory symptoms (numbness or tingling)
6. Radiation below the knee
7. Any sudden changes in the nature of pain
8. What impact on activities of daily living it has
9. Any suicidal intent and enquiry about protective factors   (5)

C. **How would you assess the impact the pain is having on his life?** (4 marks)

1. Assessment of mood
2. Ask about sleep pattern
3. Enquire about the ability to do daily activities
4. Identify whether leisure/social activities are curtailed
5. Ask about absence from work
6. Ask about social contact with family and friends
7. Coping skills, excess alcohol, or drug use (4)

D. **What other aspects of his life may affect his pain?** (3 marks)

1. Anxiety or depression, particularly if unstable
2. Concurrent stressors or major life events (physical or psychological such as bereavement, car crash, house move, divorce)
3. Employment worries (is manager supportive, financial loss, compensation, job loss, or adaptation to lighter duties)
4. Future and financial worries
5. Actions and responses of family and friends and illness-related behaviour (3)

E. **What pharmacological therapies would you recommend?** (2 marks)

1. Paracetamol or aspirin (simple analgesics)
2. NSAIDs or COX 2 inhibitors if tolerated and not contraindicated
3. Amitriptyline (particularly if sleep is problematic, but note no longer recommended by the National Institute for Health and Care Excellence (NICE)) (2)

Note: Do not recommend opioids, gabapentinoids, antidepressants, acupuncture, injections, or epidural steroids.

F. **Give 5 non-pharmacological therapies that may be useful** (5 marks)

1. Pain physiotherapy; graded exercise, pacing of activities
2. Relaxation and mindfulness techniques
3. Heat
4. TENS machine
5. Community support groups
6. Weight loss
7. Psychology: ACT (acceptance and commitment therapy)
8. Radiofrequency treatment to facet joints (5)

Total 20 marks

Further reading

NICE Guideline 59; Low back pain and sciatica in over 16s updated September 2020 https://www.nice.org.uk/guidance/ng59/chapter/Recommendations

NICE Guideline 173; Pharmacological management of neuropathic pain in non-specialist setting, updated April 2018 https://www.nice.org.uk/guidance/cg173

Question 7

A 42-year-old man presents for a nephrectomy. He is known to have dilated cardiomyopathy (DCM).

A. **Describe the pathophysiology of evolving DCM** (2 marks)

1. There is a progressive enlargement of one or both ventricles leading to reduced stroke volume
2. The dilated ventricles have low wall thickness to diameter ratio leading to increased wall stress, increased oxygen demand causing further systolic dysfunction
3. Ultimately leads to severe heart failure   (2)

B. **What are the clinical features of DCM?** (4 marks)

1. Early stages may be asymptomatic
2. Signs of heart failure—dyspnoea, fatigue, ascites, peripheral oedema, tachycardia
3. Arrhythmia
4. Embolic events
5. Sudden death   (4)

C. **List 2 of the commonest causes of DCM in the UK** (2 marks)

1. Idiopathic
2. Familial association
3. Postviral infection
4. Secondary to ischaemic heart disease or hypertension
5. Alcohol excess
6. Secondary to cardiotoxic drugs (e.g. chemotherapy or illicit drugs)
7. Neuromuscular disorder   (2)

D. List 3 classes of drug, each with an example, that are used in the medical management of DCM (6 marks)

Drug class (3 marks)	**Example** (3 marks)
1. ACE inhibitor/angiotensin 2 receptor antagonist	1. Ramipril/losartan
2. Beta-blocker	2. Bisoprolol, carvedilol
3. Loop diuretic	3. Furosemide
4. Aldosterone Inhibitor	4. Spironolactone
5. Anticoagulant (If ejection fraction ≤ 30%)	5. Aspirin, apixaban (NOAC)

(6)

E. List 2 non-pharmacological options to manage advanced heart failure secondary to DCM (2 marks)

1. Partial left ventriculotomy
2. Left ventricular assist device
3. Implantable cardioverter defibrillator device
4. Cardiac transplantation

(2)

F. The patient presents for his nephrectomy

List the cardiovascular goals when anaesthetising this patient (4 marks)

1. Avoid myocardial depression
2. Avoid tachycardia
3. Maintain preload
4. Prevent increases in afterload
5. Prevent sudden hypotension by careful titration of anaesthetic agents

(4)

Total 20 marks

Further reading

IR Ibrahim, V Sharma; Cardiomyopathy and anaesthesia, *BJA Education*, Volume 17, Issue 11, November 2017, Pages 363–369.

Question 8

A 39-year-old man is unconscious in the ED. He was pulled from a house fire by the emergency services. He has a past medical history of schizophrenia and alcohol excess. On examination the man has burns to his torso and legs amounting to 30% total body surface area. He weighs 80kg. There is no evidence of significant trauma on the primary survey.

A. State the Parkland formula, calculate his resuscitation fluid requirements for the initial 24 hours and state how this is administered (4 marks).

Parkland formula

4ml × % TBSA burn × weight in kg = mls fluid required in first 24 hours (1 mark)

1. $4 \times 30 \times 80 = 9,600$ml of crystalloid (1 mark)
2. One half of this volume = 4,800ml to be given in the first 8 hours (1 mark)
3. Second half of this volume = 4,800ml to be given in the following 16 hours (1 mark)   (4)

Note: This result is only a guide and response to fluid should be continually assessed. More fluid is likely to be needed in the event of trauma or significant airway injury. The question only asks for resuscitation fluid—maintenance fluid will be required additionally to the resuscitation volumes for the time period stated.

B. What aspects of the history from the paramedics would be associated with an increased risk of smoke inhalation injury? (2 marks)

1. Fire in an enclosed space
2. Loss of consciousness at the scene (e.g. secondary to trauma, alcohol, drugs, or hypoxia)
3. Other fatalities (indicates a higher risk of significant injuries)   (2)

C. What are the signs and symptoms of smoke inhalation injury? (6 marks)

1. Voice changes, hoarseness, stridor
2. Cough
3. Facial or airway burns
4. Soot in sputum, nose, or mouth
5. Respiratory distress
6. Reduced conscious level, confusion, or agitation
7. Clinical hypoxia, oxygen saturations <94%
8. Increased carboxyhaemoglobin on blood gas   (6)

D. This patient remains GCS 5. He has no obvious facial burns or swelling. His PaO_2 is 11kPa on 15L oxygen via a trauma mask and his carboxyhaemoglobin level is 20%. You plan to intubate the patient.

What differences and potential challenges must you be aware of when compared with a standard rapid sequence induction? (6 marks)

1. If unable to rule out cervical spine injury, manual in-line stabilization may be required
2. Have smaller diameter *uncut* ET tubes prepared as he may develop airway oedema
3. Have intravenous fluids running and vasopressors prepared and attached; induction may cause cardiovascular instability
4. Intubate with a low-pressure cuff tube
5. Anticipate difficulties and have an initial and rescue plan—potentially front of neck access
6. Check ET position with capnography, chest auscultation, and secure carefully
7. Have senior anaesthetic help immediately available
8. CXR post intubation essential   (6)

E. What 2 findings on his arterial blood gases and U&Es would suggest significant cyanide poisoning? (2 marks)

1. Elevated lactate >7mmol/L despite adequate fluid resuscitation
2. High anion gap acidosis   (2)

Total 20 marks

Further reading

S Bishop, S Maguire; Anaesthesia and intensive care for major burns, *Continuing Education in Anaesthesia Critical Care & Pain*, Volume 12, Issue 3, June 2012, Pages 118–122.

P Gill, RV Martin; Smoke inhalation injury, *Continuing Education in Anaesthesia Critical Care & Pain*, Volume 15, Issue 3, June 2015, Pages 143–148.

Question 9

You anaesthetise a 29-year-old man for urgent appendicectomy. He is ASA1 and has had a previous anaesthetic for ORIF right wrist with no problems. You perform a rapid sequence induction uneventfully with propofol and suxamethonium. Five minutes after knife to skin you note his $etCO_2$ has increased to 9kPa and his heart rate is 121 bpm. You suspect MH.

A. List 5 other potential differential diagnoses (5 marks)

1. Inadequate anaesthesia/analgesia
2. Inappropriate breathing circuit/fresh gas flow too low/erroneous ventilation settings
3. Soda lime exhausted
4. Sepsis
5. Endocrine disorder (e.g. phaeochromocytoma or thyroid crisis)
6. Neuroleptic malignant syndrome

7. Undeclared ecstasy or other recreational drug use
8. Anaphylaxis

Note: Must have the first 2 points included for all marks

B. On re-assessment his blood pressure is 81/45mmHg, his heart rate is 130bpm. His core temperature is 39.8°C and his etCO$_2$ is now 9.8kPa.

List 5 additional clinical signs that would indicate a classical MH presentation (5 marks)

1. Unexplained increase in oxygen requirements/desaturation
2. Generalized muscle rigidity
3. Myoglobinuria and increased creatine kinase
4. Cardiac arrythmias
5. Disseminated intravascular coagulopathy
6. Hyperkalaemia
7. Respiratory and metabolic acidosis   (5)

C. You declare a critical incident, halt surgery, and call for help.

Outline your acute management to halt the MH process (6 marks)
1. Discontinue inhalational agent and suxamethonium
2. Disconnect vaporizer or use a clean breathing system and anaesthetic machine
3. Hyperventilate with 100% oxygen (2–3 × minute volume at high flow rate)
4. Insert MH filters into breathing system
5. Maintain anaesthesia using propofol
6. Give dantrolene 2–3mg/kg bolus
7. Repeat boluses dantrolene 1mg/kg up to a maximum of 10mg/kg until stable
8. Commence active cooling

Note: No marks given for monitoring measures or treatment of complications of MH   (6)

D. Outline the aetiology of MH (3 marks)

1. MH susceptibility is inherited as an autosomal dominant condition with variable penetrance
2. Administration of triggering agents leads to an uncontrolled release of free calcium from the sarcoplasmic reticulum of skeletal muscle
3. This could be due to an abnormality at any point in the excitation-contraction coupling mechanism
4. The most likely site is the junction between the T tubule (involving the dihydropyridine receptor) and the sarcoplasmic reticulum (involving the ryanodine receptor, responsible for calcium efflux)   (3)

E. What is the mechanism of action of dantrolene? (1 mark)

Dantrolene is a hydantoin derivative which acts within the muscle cell to reduce calcium release by the sarcoplasmic reticulum   (1)

Total 20 marks

Further reading

Association of Anaesthetists; Malignant hyperthermia crisis 2011 https://www.aagbi.org/publications/publications-guidelines/malignant-hyperthermia-crisis

Question 10

A 6-year-old 20kg boy has sustained an open eye injury with associated threat of sight loss. He requires urgent examination under anaesthesia.

A. Describe the mechanism of further sight loss following the primary open eye injury, preoperatively? (2 marks)

1. Pain, eye rubbing, crying, breath holding, posture, coughing, vomiting, or Valsalva manoeuvres may increase intraocular pressure
2. Increased intraocular pressure may cause vitreous extrusion, haemorrhage, or lens prolapse via an open eye (2)

B. Complete the table regarding the influence of anaesthetic factors on intraocular pressure (5 marks)

Factor	Influence on IOP	Mechanism
15° head-up tilt (1 mark)	Decreased	Assists venous drainage
IV induction agent (1 mark)	Decreased	Mainly by reduction in arterial and venous blood pressures (except ketamine)
Depolarizing muscle relaxant (1 mark)	Increased	Increased tone of extraocular muscles
Laryngoscopy (1 mark)	Increased	Either pressor response or straining in an inadequately relaxed patient
Hypocapnia (pCO_2 3.5–4.0kPa) (1 mark)	Decreased	Reduced blood volume by constriction of choroidal blood vessels

Note: Need both answers correct in each row to award one mark (5)

C. Following commencement of the procedure in theatre, the patient develops severe bradycardia. Describe the oculocardiac reflex arc by completing the table (7 marks)

Trigger (1 mark)	1. Traction on extraocular muscles and/or globe pressure
Afferent arc (2 marks)	1. Fibres running with long and short ciliary nerves 2. Via trigeminal (CN V) ganglion near floor of 4th ventricle
Efferent arc (2 marks)	1. By Vagus nerve (CN X) 2. Fibres to the medulla (respiratory and vomiting centre) 3. By Vagus nerve to sino-atrial node
Effects (2 marks)	1. Bradycardia 2. Reduction in breathing 3. Nausea/vomiting

(7)

D. The surgeon begins to examine the child under anaesthetic. The heart rate drops to 21 beats per minute.

Outline in detail the immediate management (3 marks)

1. Ask surgeon to cease activity
2. Administer atropine 20mcg/kg = 400mcg (or 0.4mg)
3. Lift arm/deliver flush via fluid bolus
4. Commence CPR

Note: Answer asks for detail—must state dose of atropine for full marks (3)

E. Briefly describe 3 ways to further reduce the likelihood of adverse oculomedullary reflexes in this case? (3 marks)

1. Use of local anaesthetic block (abolishes afferent arc)
2. Avoiding hypocapnia (which sensitizes the reflex)
3. Prophylactic administration of antimuscarinic (e.g. glycopyrrolate or atropine)
4. Gentle surgical technique (3)

Total 20 marks

Further reading

H Murgatroyd, J Bembridge; Intraocular pressure, *Continuing Education in Anaesthesia Critical Care & Pain*, Volume 8, Issue 3, 2008, Pages 100–103.

Question 11

A 74-year-old man presents for an elective triple vessel coronary artery bypass.

A. List 6 patient related factors that are used in the European System for Cardiac Operative Risk Evaluation (EUROScore2) (6 marks)

1. Age >60
2. Female sex
3. Chronic obstructive pulmonary disease (COPD)
4. Extracardiac arteriopathy
5. Neurological dysfunction or disease
6. Previous cardiac surgery
7. Raised serum creatinine
8. Active endocarditis
9. Critical preoperative state (e.g. history of ventricular fibrillation (VF) or pulseless ventricular tachycardia (VT), required preoperative ventilation, cardiac massage, or intra-aortic balloon pump)

Note: No marks given for operative or specific cardiac risk factors (6)

B. The surgeon is performing the operation on cardiopulmonary bypass.

List 6 components of a basic cardiopulmonary bypass circuit (6 marks)

1. Venous cannula
2. Reservoirs
3. Pumps
4. Membrane oxygenator
5. Heat exchanger
6. Filter
7. Arterial Cannula

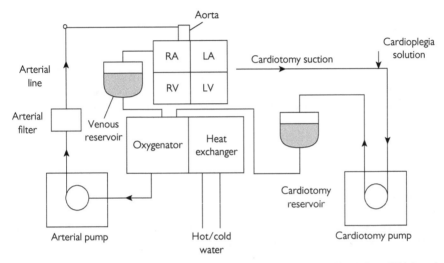

Reproduced from SAQs for the Final FRCA, Shorthouse J et al., Figure 12. Copyright Oxford University Press, 2011. Reproduced with permission of the Licensor through PLSclear.

(6)

C. List 2 functions of cardioplegia in cardiac surgery (2 marks)

1. To produce diastolic arrest and a motionless field for the surgeon.
2. Myocardial protection
3. H+ ion buffering
4. Free radical scavenging
5. Reduce myocardial oedema
6. Improve microvascular flow

Also, addition of specific substances (e.g. aspartate and glutamate can promote oxidative metabolism in an energy depleted heart)

(2)

D. The surgery proceeds uneventfully using cardiopulmonary bypass and hypothermia. Outline your preparation in anticipation of weaning this patient from cardiopulmonary bypass (6 marks)

1. Re-warm to a core temperature >36°C
2. Measure and correct metabolic abnormalities (e.g. acidosis or hyperkalaemia)
3. Treat hyperglycaemia
4. Ensure haemoglobin >70g/L
5. Correct coagulation abnormalities
6. Ensure in sinus rhythm with rate controlled
7. Ventilate and preoxygenate with 100% oxygen
8. Confirm de-airing of the heart and great vessels with TOE
9. Have all emergency drugs and equipment ready   (6)

Total 20 marks

Further reading

T Scott, J Swanevelder; Perioperative myocardial protection, *Continuing Education in Anaesthesia Critical Care & Pain*, Volume 9, Issue 3, June 2009, Pages 97–101.

European System for Cardiac Operative Risk Evaluation (Euroscore) http://www.euroscore.org/

Question 12

A 54-year-old male patient is listed as an emergency to receive cadaveric renal transplantation. He has end-stage renal failure maintained on haemodialysis.

A. List 4 of the most common primary causes of end stage renal failure in the UK? (4 marks)

1. Diabetes mellitus
2. Glomerulonephritis
3. Hypertension
4. Polycystic kidney disease
5. Pyelonephritis
6. Renal vascular disease   (4)

B. How is CKD classified? (2 marks)

1. Classified using glomerular filtration rate (GFR) depending on the extent of failure: G1–G5
2. Classified using albumin to creatinine ratio (ACR): A1–A3   (2)

Note: classification of chronic renal failure uses a combination of both these scales together to fully classify as per NICE guidance (e.g. a patient might be described as G4A2)

C. **What factors inform the assessment of this patient's dialysis dependency preoperatively?** (5 marks)

1. Frequency and duration of dialysis (usually for several hours 3–4 times per week)
2. Dialysis via line or fistula
3. Volume usually removed per session
4. Any current daily fluid restriction in place
5. Patient's native urine output daily
6. Acid base status
7. Electrolyte balance (5)

D. **What are the indications for dialysis before transplantation?** (3 marks)

1. Hyperkalaemia
2. Fluid overload
3. Uraemia
4. Acidosis (3)

E. **What potential problems are presented by recent dialysis if proceeding to surgery immediately after its completion?** (2 marks)

1. Intravascular depletion/hypovolaemia
2. Possible residual anticoagulation (2)

F. **The patient has a functional AVF in his right forearm.**

How should the AVF sites be protected intraoperatively? (4 marks)
1. Avoid cannulating the AVF limb
2. Avoid non-invasive blood pressure on the AVF arm
3. Wrap it in padding/cotton wool
4. Careful positioning/monitoring of the arm to present traction or compression injuries
5. Preference to cannulate the dorsum only, of the (other) hand to avoid future AVF sites of forearm and antecubital veins
6. Restricting use of arterial lines to essential only, with the radial site preferred (4)

Total 20 marks

Further reading

T Bradley, T Teare, Q Milner; Anaesthetic management of patients requiring vascular access surgery for renal dialysis. *BJA Education*, Volume 17, Issue 8, 2017, Pages 269–274.

D Mayhew, D Ridgway, JM Hunter; Update on the intraoperative management of adult cadaveric renal transplantation. *BJA Education*, Volume 16, Issue 2, 2016, Pages 53–57.

National Institute for Health and Clinical Excellence (NICE); Chronic kidney disease in adults: assessment and management 2014 https://www.nice.org.uk/guidance/cg182

Appendix 1

Some candidates may prefer to examine individual curriculum topics to supplement their private study instead of undertaking the variety of an exam paper. Listed below are the questions grouped together by topic theme. They are described in the format 'Paper Number-Question Number' i.e. paper 1, question number 2 is denoted as 1-2. Some questions have multiple topics. The advanced sciences are represented more generally within all of the questions.

General duties

Airway management

   1-12, 3-3, 4-8, 5-7, 5-11

Critical incidents

   2-5, 4-3, 4-9, 6-9, 6-10

Day surgery

   1-4

General, urological, and gynaecological surgery

   1-3, 2-1, 3-5, 3-12, 4-3, 4-6, 4-11, 5-2, 6-7, 6-9, 6-12

Ear, nose, throat (ENT), maxillofacial, and dental surgery

   1-12, 2-4, 3-3, 3-11, 4-8, 5-6, 5-7

Management of respiratory and cardiac arrest

   4-3, 6-10

Non-theatre

   1-6, 5-9

Orthopaedic surgery

   1-11, 2.9, 3-9, 4-9, 5-12, 6-2

Perioperative medicine

   1-7, 2-1, 2-4, 2-7, 2-8, 2-9, 3-1, 3-9, 3-12, 4-1, 5-3, 6-3

Regional anaesthesia

   1-11, 2-6, 3-6, 4-9, 4-12, 5-1

Sedation

   3-3

Transfer medicine

   5-9

Trauma and stabilisation

   2-11, 3-8

Mandatory units

Anaesthesia for neurosurgery, neuroradiology, and neurocritical care

1-5, 2-11, 3-1, 3-4, 3-8, 4-11, 5-5

Cardiothoracic anaesthesia and cardiothoracic critical care

1-8, 2-7, 4-1, 5-3, 6-7, 6-11

Intensive care medicine

1-2, 2-2, 2-9, 2-11, 3-4, 3-7, 3-8, 4-4, 5-8, 5-11, 6-8

Obstetric anaesthesia

1-1, 2-12, 3-10, 4-10, 5-4, 6-1, 6-4

Paediatric anaesthesia

1-10, 2-2, 3-11, 4-2, 5-7, 5-10, 5-11, 6-10

Pain medicine

1-9, 2-3, 2-6, 2-10, 4-5, 6-1, 6-6

Optional units

Ophthalmic anaesthesia

4-12, 4-2, 6-10

Plastics and burns

3-2, 6-8

Vascular surgery anaesthesia

2-6, 5-1, 6-5, 6-12

Index

Notes: Page numbers in *q* refer to Question and *a* refer to Answer.